The Geriatric Patient

Considerations and Strategies for Safe, Effective Care

Joint Commission Resources

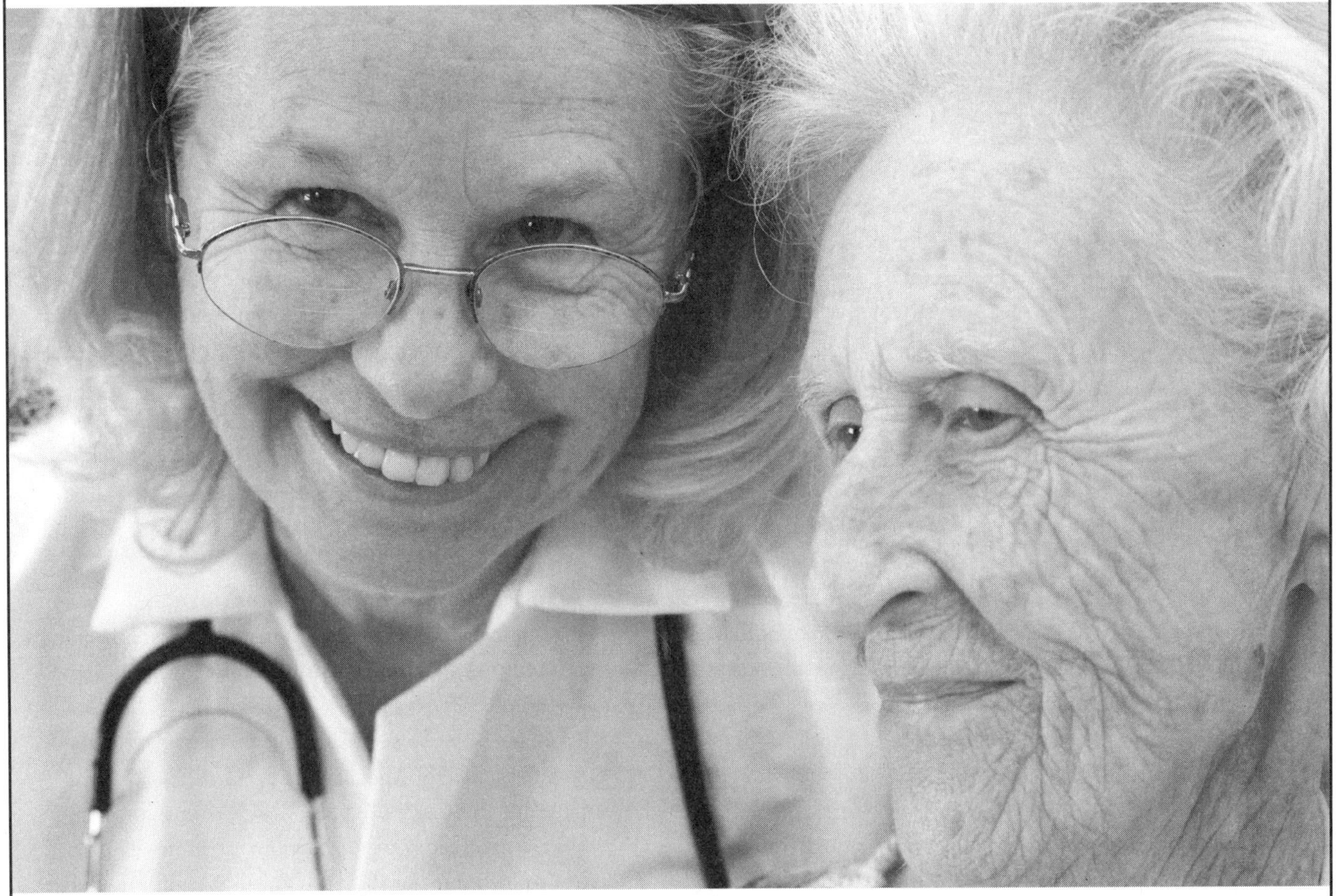

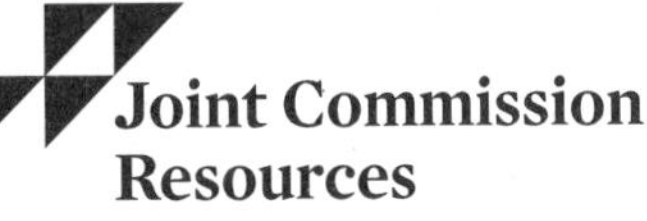

Senior Editor: **Audrie Bretl Roelf, M.A.**
Project Manager: **Christine Wyllie, M.A.**
Manager, Publications: **Paul Reis**
Associate Director, Production: **Johanna Harris**
Associate Director, Editorial Development: **Diane Bell**
Executive Director: **Catherine Chopp Hinckley, Ph.D.**
Vice President, Learning: **Charles J. Macfarlane, F.A.C.H.E.**
Joint Commission/JCR Reviewers: **Diane Bell, Elaine Buccellato, John Fishbeck, Nancy Gorman, Peggy Lavin, Cynthia Leslie, Paul Reis, Paul vanOstenberg, Debra Zak**

Joint Commission Resources Mission

The mission of Joint Commission Resources (JCR) is to continuously improve the safety and quality of health care in the United States and in the international community through the provision of education, publications, consultation, and evaluation services.

Joint Commission Resources educational programs and publications support, but are separate from, the accreditation activities of The Joint Commission. Attendees at Joint Commission Resources educational programs and purchasers of Joint Commission Resources publications receive no special consideration or treatment in, or confidential information about, the accreditation process.

The inclusion of an organization name, product, or service in a Joint Commission Resources publication should not be construed as an endorsement of such organization, product, or service, nor is failure to include an organization name, product, or service to be construed as disapproval.

This publication is designed to provide accurate and authoritative information in regard to the subject matter covered. Every attempt has been made to ensure accuracy at the time of publication; however, please note that laws, regulations, and standards are subject to change. Please also note that some of the examples in this publication are specific to the laws and regulations of the locality of the facility. The information and examples in this publication are provided with the understanding that the publisher is not engaged in providing medical, legal, or other professional advice. If any such assistance is desired, the services of a competent professional person should be sought.

Joint Commission Resources, Inc. (JCR), a not-for-profit affiliate of The Joint Commission, has been designated by The Joint Commission to publish publications and multimedia products. JCR reproduces and distributes these materials under license from The Joint Commission.

Printed in the U.S.A. 5 4 3 2 1

ISBN: 978-1-59940-316-8
Library of Congress Control Number: 2009925352

For more information about Joint Commission Resources, please visit http://www.jcrinc.com.

Contents

Foreword

Caring for the Geriatric Patient: *A Unique Challenge*

Paul vanOstenberg, D.D.S., M.S.,
International Accreditation and Standards,
Joint Commission International

Statistics from most countries around the world demonstrate the aging of populations. While this fact presents a variety of demographic, social, and financial challenges for these countries, the impact on the health care systems is most profound in terms of meeting the needs of those with long-standing chronic conditions, increasing dependency, and decreasing personal and financial resources. It is becoming more common to see an older patient confused and clutching a bag of medications in a hospital's emergency department. This may not be true in all countries, as social support systems vary; payment mechanisms vary from universal coverage to 100% out of pocket; and the family unit may be either tight and intact or fragmented, with the older adult living in congregate or sheltered settings distant from families.

The worldwide patient safety movement has put a face on the quality movement; however, that face has been generic until recently, when the safety issues for children and geriatric patients began to be more clearly identified. It was natural for these two groups to come to the forefront together, as the old and the young present many of the same parameters that make patient safety unique and complex. Both groups have limited independent decision-making capacity, are heavily dependent on family and others to facilitate the care process, have unique learning needs and capacities, and frequently have complex health care needs. Add to this the rapid and highly complex health care process, new technologies, and fragmentation of care settings, and it is no wonder patient safety events are common. In fact, what is surprising is that adverse safety events are not more common.

The health professions have come a long way in identifying the unique knowledge and skills of those who care for the aged population. These professions recognize that age alone does not determine disability and dependence—there is a significant group of older adults who are vigorous and articulate patients. These professionals also recognize the differences between normal and abnormal aging and how to engage the family and others in the care process—unfortunately, sometimes unnecessarily marginalizing the older patient. Applying this unique knowledge and skill set is often difficult, as the health care system most frequently segments patients by disease and diagnosis rather than by age. Thus, all health professionals, both those with and without the unique knowledge and skill set, end up caring for geriatric patients.

Thus, there is a need for all health professionals to be reminded periodically of the primary accommodations needed to care for the aged and, in particular, how predominate characteristics of the aged may contribute to adverse or even sentinel patient safety events. This book is that needed periodic review of the common and uncommon that can make the care of the aged safer. While the focus of this book is on the aged, the skills and knowledge are applicable to all patient care and grounded in the patient safety movement.

A simple and often repeated saying is: Treat all patients as if they were your aged parents or as if you were the patient and that age—simple logic but a real-life daily challenge.

Introduction

In its 2002 publication *Active Aging: A Policy Framework,* the World Health Organization (WHO) announced that population aging is a challenge to society. The very fact that our population is aging and able to look forward to an increasing life expectancy is welcome news, but it does present a challenge for which health care organizations need to prepare. The older adult population is growing rapidly. In the decades to come, those over the age of 65 will represent a vast proportion of the overall global population. In the United States alone, it is estimated that in the year 2030, 20% of the population—also known as the "baby boomers"—will be age 65 or older.[1] According to the U.S. Census Bureau, the age 85 and older population is expected to more than triple over the next several decades, from 5.4 million to 19 million by 2050.

On a global scale, there are similar figures to consider. While current data points to the fact that the growth in older adult populations is being seen more in developed countries in the "Global North," aging is a worldwide phenomenon. A United Nations study on global aging predicts that by 2050, 21% of the global population will be age 60 and over. Even the median age of the global population is impacted by aging; the worldwide median age is 26, but this is not represented in individual countries, particularly those who are facing a growing older adult population. Consider, for example, a country such as Japan that has a median age of 41 or Spain that is predicted to have a median age of 55 by 2050.[2]

On the one hand, the news of a global population that is enjoying greater longevity is a welcome one, because it points to improvements in the quality of life that are extending life expectancy; but on the other, it also has implications for health care organizations. The current older adult population represents approximately 12.5% of the current U.S. population, but it accounts for approximately 60% of hospital admissions.[3] The older adult population also accounts for 48% of hospital days, 65% of all hospital discharges for heart disease, 55% of discharges for malignant neoplasms, 90% of discharges for strokes, and 46% of patients in critical care for a variety of reasons.[4] Fully 69% of patients receiving home care in the United States are aged 65 and older.[5] In the United States, approximately 1.5 million residents currently receive long term care, and 955,000 patients receive home care.[6] With a growing aging population, these trends and developments, often those that put strain on a health care organization's resources, are likely to be on the rise.

In the preface to the Institute of Medicine's 2008 report *Retooling for an Aging America: Building the Health Care Workforce,* John Rowe, M.D., outlines some of the biggest challenges that health care organizations face as the population ages.

> Caring for the elderly population poses a unique set of challenges. In addition to geriatric syndromes, such as falls and malnutrition, which often lead to acute health care problems, older adults also suffer from a range of cognitive impairments that can impact their ability to perform as active participants in their own care.
>
> The health care workforce in general receives very little geriatric training and is not prepared to deliver the best care to older patients.

> . . . Since virtually all health care workers care for older adults to some degree, the geriatric competence of all providers must also be improved more generally, through significant enhancements in educational curricula and training programs.[7]

The concern over the health care industry's ability to care and plan for the rise in older adult patients, referred to as the "silver tsunami," is not a new one.

Health care leaders are stressing the alarming lack of a coordinated or strategic response to this unavoidable change in global demographics, a change that will have a dramatic impact on health care organizations. With their complicated medical histories and conditions, special needs, complex combination of prescribed medications to treat a variety of conditions, and high risks for such things as falls or pressure ulcers, caring for older adult patients requires specialized training and experience.[8] And these are specialized skills that not all health care workers readily have. Many are being asked or expected to adapt.

Based on these staggering numbers, the health care industry immediately needs to address concerns related to the care and treatment of older adult patients and do so in creative ways. Adding more qualified staff to an organization may not be the only (or the best) solution. Like other special populations, older adult patients face special challenges that require a special approach to their care to ensure their safety. It is not uncommon for geriatric patients to navigate the health care system with a complex array of medical concerns. They may have a chronic illness, be more frail, and be taking multiple medications, for example. Each of these conditions alone can make care more complex, but when patients have a combination of these conditions, the complexity increases, making ensuring their safety an even larger issue. Are health care organizations prepared? Are their staff trained and educated to cope with the special needs that older adult patients can face? Have organizations considered what an increase in the number of geriatric patients might mean for how they function and deliver care? Are they putting systems and processes in place to ensure that older adult patients are safe and do not experience any adverse events?

A common concern for older adult patients is cascade iatrogenesis, which is when a patient has a medical or nursing intervention that sets off a sequence of adverse events that leads to a decline in that patient's status. This has been found to happen most often in the oldest, most functionally impaired patients who are sickest on admission.[9]

Older adult patients have the same needs as any other patient population while in a health care organization: They need to receive high-quality, safe care. And as with all patients, they can be vulnerable to medication errors, wrong-site surgery, health care–acquired infections, and other hazards. In addition, other common risks that can result in adverse events for older adult patients include falls, pressure ulcers, abuse and neglect, mental health and memory concerns, polypharmacy, and many others.

About This Book

This book will help leaders of health care organizations, especially hospitals, home care organizations, and ambulatory care and long term care facilities—anywhere older adult patients are treated—consider those crucial issues in preparation for an aging population. This book highlights the key points and issues relating to older adult patient safety and provides strategies, case studies, and tips aimed at helping health care organizations address the following quality and patient safety issues specifically concerning older adult patients:

- Communication
- Infection control
- Medication safety
- Environment of care
- Memory and mental status
- Suicide risk
- Nutrition and hydration
- Fall prevention
- Skin care and pressure ulcers

It should be noted that *The Geriatric Patient: Considerations and Strategies for Safe, Effective Care* is not intended for health care organizations in the United States alone. Although each country may have its own unique challenges and concerns in relation to older adult patient safety, as was earlier noted, aging is a growing international concern, particularly in the "Global North" or in developed countries, and this trend shows no sign of slowing. All health care organizations and systems, regardless of their geographic location, need to prepare and plan for the care of their growing older adult patient population. The tips and strategies included in this publication can provide all health care organizations with helpful guidance on ensuring that their older adult patients are safe.

As a result, the publication has attempted to include as much data and statistics as possible from beyond the borders of the United States. There are some cases, however, where the only data available is U.S. specific. In those cases, health care organizations from beyond the United States should still consider the U.S. data in their own planning and improvement activities. Global studies into older adult health and aging are underway, however. In 2005, the WHO announced that it is undertaking a large-scale Study on Global AGEing and Adult Health (SAGE), which is part of a survey program aimed at compiling comprehensive longitudinal information on the health and well-being of adult populations. This study is being conducted in countries around the world, and information on it and its forthcoming publication of findings are and will be available at http://www.who.int/healthinfo/systems/sage/en/index.html.

The Geriatric Patient: Considerations and Strategies for Safe, Effective Care includes the following elements:

Chapter 1: Communication and Older Adults discusses the importance of clear and well-functioning communication in the care and safety of older adult patients. It includes a discussion of provider-provider and provider-patient communication.

Chapter 2: Improving the Physical Environment for Older Adults looks at the environment of care risk factors that can increase the risk of harm to older adult patients.

Chapter 3: Medication Safety for Older Adults considers the problems of polypharmacy, medication nonadherence, and adverse drug events in older adult patient safety. It also looks at the use of technology to improve medication safety.

Chapter 4: Infection Control Issues for Older Adults discusses the infection control risks that organizations should consider when planning for older adult patient safety.

Chapter 5: Fall Prevention and Older Adults with falls being a major patient safety risk for older adult patients, discusses ways for organizations to prevent falls. It also includes a case study.

Chapter 6: Memory, Mental Health Issues, and Older Adults looks at risk associated with depression, dementia, and suicide risk among older adult patients.

Chapter 7: Spotting Abuse or Neglect in Older Adults considers how organizations can work to assess and intervene to reduce the incidence of abuse or neglect in older adult patients.

Chapter 8: Special Needs and Older Adults discusses how organizations can prepare for special issues that older adult patients are particularly challenged by, such as pressure ulcers, incontinence, and skin problems.

Terms Used

Because this book is intended to address a variety of patient safety risks that affect the elderly in different health care settings, the publication has employed the use of the terms "older adults" or "older adult patient" to refer to any elderly, aging, or geriatric individual, client, resident, or patient receiving care, treatment, and services in any type of health care organization, including home care, ambulatory care, long term care, and hospitals. In those instances where an example is more specific, such as in the case of a description of a resident in a long term care facility, the publication will employ language that is more specific to that type of health care setting. Although some of the strategies or issues raised in this publication may not be applicable in certain states or countries, aspects of what is shared can be applied to different locations and settings for the benefit of health care organizations.

Acknowledgments

Joint Commission Resources (JCR) relies on the insight, perspective, and experiences of many individuals and organizations to help shape and contribute to its publications. JCR would like to thank all the reviewers and content experts at The Joint Commission and JCR who helped conceptualize and develop the book's topics. It would also like to thank Pocono Medical Center, VNA Hospice of Monroe County, and Poudre Valley Hospital for their generous willingness to be profiled in this publication about their efforts to improve older adult patient safety. JCR is also grateful to Elaine Buccellato, R.N., B.S.N., M.S., for her insights into older adult patient safety, which are interspersed throughout this work. A special thanks goes out to Ladan Cockshut for her talent and diligence in writing this book.

References

1. He W. et al.: *65+ in the United States: Current population report.* U.S. Census Bureau, Washington, DC: U.S. Government Printing Office, 2005.
2. Kinsella K., Velkoff V.A.: U.S. Census Bureau Series P95/01-1, *An Aging World: 2001,* U.S. Government Printing Office, Washington, DC, 2001. http://www.census.gov/prod/2001pubs/p95-01-1.pdf (accessed Mar. 18, 2009).
3. DeFrances C.J., Hall M.J.: *2002 Discharge National Hospital Discharge Survey. Advance data from vital and health statistics* (No. 342). Hyattsville, MD: National Center for Health Statistics, 2004.
4. O'Neill G., Barry P.: *Training physicians in geriatric care: Responding to critical need.* 2003. http://www.agingsociety.org/agingsociety/pdf/trainging.pdf (accessed Feb. 19, 2009).
5. National Association for Home Care and Hospice: *Basic Statistics about Home Care.* Updated 2008. http://www.nahc.org/facts/08HC_Stats.pdf. (accessed Mar. 18, 2009).
6. National Center for Health Statistics: *Health, United States, 2007 with Chartbook on Trends in the Health of Americans.* Hyattsville, MD: National Center for Health Statistics, 2007. http://www.cdc.gov/nchs/data/hus/hus07.pdf#104. (accessed Mar. 18, 2009).
7. Committee on the Future Health Care Workforce for Older Americans, Institute of Medicine: *Retooling for an Aging America: Building the Health Care Workforce.* Washington, DC: National Academies, 2008.
8. Lewis R.C.: Medical schools prepare for "silver tsunami." http://www.reuters.com/article/latestCrisis/idUSN28499322 (accessed Feb. 19, 2009).
9. Hartford Institute for Geriatric Nursing: Want to know more: iatrogenesis. http://www.consultgerirn.org/topics/iatrogenesis/want_to_know_more (accessed Feb. 19, 2009).

Chapter 1

Communication and Older Adults

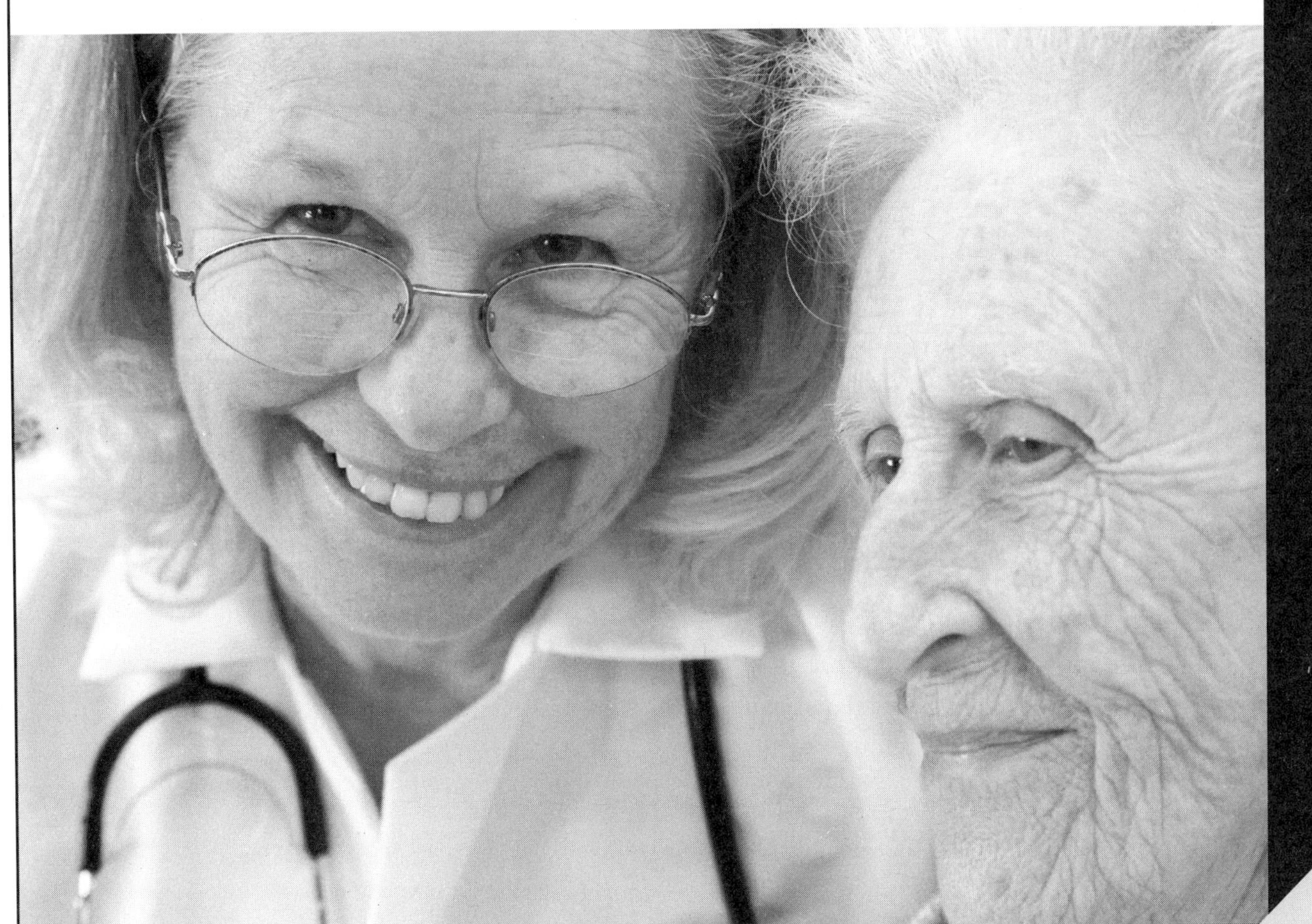

Older Adult Patient Safety and Communication: An Important Link

Effective communication is a key element of a patient's satisfaction with his or her care experience and is a crucial contributing factor to an organization's ability to provide safe, high-quality care. In the case of older adult patients, communication is especially important. Even how staff communicate with an older adult patient may require special training and consideration.

It is fitting that the first chapter of this publication begins with a discussion of what can often be viewed as a fundamental aspect of ensuring patient safety: good communication. Often cited as a root cause of sentinel events, poor communication can have disastrous results for an organization wanting to deliver high-quality, safe care to its patients. Communication is not merely an issue that relates to how a health care organization communicates with its patients—it also relates to how staff members communicate among themselves, with other organizations, and with patients and their families. Considering the complex needs and concerns that can impact an older adult patient, organizations must work to ensure that all forms of communication work well on all levels. This applies to everything from policies and procedures, initial contact with a patient, assessment, medication reconciliation, care planning, staff interaction and communication, patient and family education, communication with external agencies and departments, handoff communication, discharge planning, and so on. Many factors go into ensuring smooth and consistent communication: trained and empowered staff, well-designed policies and procedures, effective assessment and care planning processes, good teamwork skills, leadership support, and a culture of safety, to name a few. Even communication between family members—or responsible caregivers—and older adult patients can have an effect on ensuring that patient's safety.

Often the biggest errors resulting from communication between staff or health care organizations occur at those crucial milestonelike points in the care of patients, including the following:

- Assessment and/or admission
- Care planning
- Handoffs
- Discharge

Those crucial yet delicate moments in care have been found to lead to breakdowns in consistent or effective care, which can lead to adverse events for a patient. In the case of older adult patients, these moments can make them even more vulnerable to risk. How an organization designs its process and systems to communicate at these and other important milestones can make the difference between safe, ongoing care and an increased risk of adverse events.

One important consideration for health care organizations is understanding where common mistakes in communicating with patients can take place so that they can be aware of them and work toward eliminating them. Some common errors that are made in health care–related communication with patients include the following:[1]

- Writing prescription drug instructions at an eleventh-grade reading level, rather than a fifth-grade reading level
- Communicating in medical jargon when it is unnecessary
- Sending patients to the Internet for additional instructions and follow-up care
- Providing reading material in a font size that is too small
- Not using simple visuals for medical instructions
- Not recognizing that a patient may be being polite rather than expressing understanding when he or she nods or says "yes"
- Failing to demonstrate cultural awareness and sensitivity in patient encounters
- Talking too quickly and not allowing time for the patient to ask questions
- Not providing medical information in the patient's primary language
- Not taking time to explain the meaning of prescription bottle labels

In addition, research has found that additional communication errors take place when caring for older adult patients, including the following:

- Not feeling listened to or understood.[2]
- The use of "elderspeak" by staff when communicating with older adult patients.[3] Elderspeak is a kind of speech that is similar to "baby talk" and which is often lacking in respect (*see* page 14 for more information on this type of speech).
- A lack of interpersonal interaction between staff and patients.[4]
- Providing too much information or confusing instructions in relation to medication use or postdischarge care.

Notes from the Field: Communication and Older Adult Patient Safety

Elaine Buccellato, R.N., B.S.N., M.S., Joint Commission surveyor in long term care and hospital settings, states that although effective communication is vital for all patients, it is especially significant for the older adult patient and includes at least the following:

- Effective communication ascertains that the verbal and written information is appropriate to the specialized needs of the older adult patient.
- Effective communication uses the older adult patient's ability to learn and understand as a basis for communication and education.
- Effective communication validates that the older adult patient is able to comply with the instructions, if required. It also addresses any barriers to communication, such as vision, speech, hearing, motivation, or cognitive impairment.

An older adult patient may have one or many of these impairments that can impede his or her communication and ability to learn.

Therefore, effective communication and patient education are uniquely connected to ensure older adult patient safety. "You should never underestimate the importance of assessing the older adult patient's ability to learn," says Buccellato. Buccellato notes that both The Joint Commission's and The Joint Commission International's standards specify that the assessment of learning needs addresses cultural and religious beliefs, emotional barriers, desire and motivation to learn, physical or cognitive limitations, and barriers to communication as appropriate. The education should be based on the older adult patient's condition and assessed needs. Buccellato notes, "With any education strategy, it's crucial to provide it at the right time for patients. For example, education should begin on admission and as soon as the needs have been determined and not just when a patient is being discharged. Time of discharge may not be the best time to give important instructions. If you're teaching older adult patients about medications and medication safety, slow down when you're giving instructions." She also notes that giving too much information to an older adult patient too quickly could be confusing. Organizations should take time to assess and streamline their communication and teaching approaches. Evaluation of the older adult patient's comprehension and demonstrated evidence of learning are crucial to his or her safety in the health care facility and when at home.

Although this chapter does not go into comprehensive detail regarding the many elements of errors in communication and in ensuring effective communication for older adult patients, it does lay out the most pressing concerns for organizations to consider as they work toward designing systems and processes with older adult patient safety in mind.

In Notes from the Field, left, a health care expert with particular experience in the area of older adult patient safety stresses the importance of the relationship between patient safety and effective communication.

Communication Between Health Care Providers

At the core of any effective communication strategy is how well health care providers communicate with each other. How an organization communicates its policies and procedures, conducts its assessments, plans care, educates staff and patients, plans discharges, and communicates with patients and family members can have an impact on patient safety. Special consideration has to be taken for older adult patients who may have special assessment needs, particular risk factors that can impact their care and safety, or particular communication needs that should be planned for in advance. Depending on the health care setting, some staff may have limited training and experience regarding the care and assessment of older adult patients, or processes and systems may need to be put in place to ensure that certain high-risk factors are managed, such as the prevalence for pressure ulcers or falls among older adult patients.

Consider the following questions when assessing how well health care organizations communicate between each other and how staff communicate between each other:

- Does your organization have a good culture of safety?
- Does your organization data point to any particular problems relating to communication?
- During shift changes, how effectively do your staff communicate with each other?
- If there is a concern over a potential patient safety risk, does your organization have a well-functioning process for staff to communicate a concern?
- How well does your handoff process function? Have there been any near misses or adverse events related to a breakdown in handoffs?
- If you are a nonhospital setting, how well does your organization communicate with medical staff during off

hours? How well do you communicate critical test results?

Policies and Procedures

An organization's formally documented policies and procedures help frame its fundamental functioning. However, these policies and procedures do more than that. They help establish consistency and clear expectations for performance, and they also allow for the systematic integration of evidence-based practices that help ensure patient safety.

When considering communications needs of older adult patients, it is important to ensure that any policies and procedures that would impact older adult patients account for any special needs that they may have. It can be helpful to take stock of all policies and procedures that could impact the quality and safety of older adult patient care to determine if they are meeting the needs of patients served and to determine if any new policies and procedures should be designed. Consider the following particular issues when looking at your policies and procedures in relation to older adult patients:

- Are the policies and procedures designed with older adult patients' special needs in mind? Do any older adult patient–specific policies need to be included?
- What is the structure of the policy and procedure? Have key staff or leadership "walked" through the policy and procedure to verify if there are any problems with it?
- If changes are made to the policies and procedures, how will these changes be communicated to staff?
- What measures will be put in place to sustain the changes or improvements? How will progress be measured?

Figure 1-1 on pages 5–6 is an example of a policy and procedure for skin assessment and wound care from VNA Hospice of Monroe County, East Stroudsburg, Pennsylvania.

Examining Organization Data

Another way to take stock of whether current policies and procedures are serving the needs of older adult patients and encouraging effective communication among staff is to look at organization data. Has there been a rise in the incidence of patient falls or pressure ulcers? Have patient satisfaction results pointed to any breakdowns in effective communication or education, particularly as they relate to older adult patients? Does staff have sufficient training and experience with older adult patients?

Tracer Methodology

An additional method to assess how well policies and procedures are serving the needs of an organization is to use tracer methodology to trace a policy and procedure. Tracer methodology is a methodology used by The Joint Commission during its on-site survey process and has also been adopted by many health care organizations as a management tool to assess systems and processes within an organization. It traces a patient or process in an organization by literally "following" the patient's or process' movement through an organization—this is done with the express purpose of assessing how well systems and processes function within an organization to provide care, treatment, and services. In the case of a patient tracer, a patient's entire care experience is traced through an organization; in the case of a systems tracer, a process or system—such as infection control or medication management—is traced within an organization. This concept can be applied to tracing a policy and procedure by having staff literally "walk through" that policy. In the case of older adult patients, the policy should be "traced" with their special needs in mind.

Some examples of the types of policies and procedures that relate particularly to older adult patients' needs and that may need review on the part of a health care organization include the following:

- Patient falls reduction and education
- Wound care and skin assessment
- Patient education
- Medication reconciliation
- Handoff communication and transportation
- Assessments: falls risk, pressure ulcer, pain assessment, nutritional screening, and so on
- Patient education
- Discharge planning
- Mental health or cognitive function

Enforcement of Policies and Procedures

After policies and procedures relating to older adult patients are in place, they have to be followed consistently. This is important for two reasons:

1. Systematic, consistent adherence to a process reduces variability and reduces risk to patient safety.

Figure 1-1. Wound Healing Guidelines and Guidance

Wound Healing Guidelines and Guidance from the Centers for Medicare and Medicaid Services

Policy: The Centers for Medicare and Medicaid Services (CMS) has finalized guidance for clinicians regarding definitions for wound healing. The CMS has collaborated with the Wound Ostomy Continence Nurses Society (WOCN) to clarify the definitions for various stages of wound healing as described in the Outcome and Assessment Information Set (OASIS). It is the policy of the agency to follow the CMS guidelines when performing wound assessment.

Purpose: The purpose of this information policy is to clarify clinical assessments of patient wounds for classification purposes and to provide interpretive guidelines for clinicians to follow.

Terms Defined:

Pressure Ulcer: Any lesion caused by unrelieved pressure resulting in damage of underlying tissue. Pressure ulcers are located over bony prominences and are staged to classify the degree of tissue damage observed.

Pressure ulcer stages:

A. **Stage I:** Nonblanchable erythema of intact skin, the heralding lesion of skin ulceration. In darker-skinned persons, discoloration of the skin, warmth, edema, induration, or hardness may also be indicators.

B. **Stage II:** Partial thickness skin loss involving epidermis, dermis, or both. The ulcer is superficial and presents as an abrasion, blister, or shallow crater.

C. **Stage III:** Full thickness skin loss involving damage to or necrosis of subcutaneous tissue that may extend down to, but not through, underlying fascia. The ulcer presents clinically as a deep crater with or without undermining of adjacent tissue.

D. **Stage IV:** Full thickness skin loss with extensive destruction, tissue necrosis, or damage to muscle, bone, or supporting structures, such as tendons and joint capsules. Undermining and sinus tracts may also be associated with stage intravenous ulcers.

E. **Nonobservable:** The wound is *UNABLE* to be visualized due to an orthopedic device or dressing, and so on. A pressure ulcer cannot be accurately staged until the deepest viable tissue layer is visible. This means that wounds covered with *ESCHAR* and or *SLOUGH* cannot be staged and should be documented as non-observable.

Stages of healing for pressure ulcers and stasis ulcers:

A. **Fully granulating:** Wound bed filled with granulation tissue to the level of the surrounding skin or new epithelium; no dead space, no avascular tissue; no signs or symptoms of infection; wound edges are open.

B. **Early/partial granulation:** More than 25% of the wound bed is covered with granulation tissue; there is minimal avascular tissue (< 25% of the wound bed is covered with avascular tissue); may have dead space; no signs of infection; wound edges are open.

C. **Nonhealing:** Wound with more than 25% of avascular tissue *OR* signs/symptoms of infection *OR* clean but nongranulating wound bed *OR* closed/hyperkeratotic wound edges *OR* persistent failure to improve despite appropriate comprehensive wound management.

continued

The above figure is an example of a policy and procedure for skin assessment and wound care.

Source: *VNA Hospice of Monroe County, East Stroudsburg, Pennsylvania. Used with permission.*

Figure 1-1. Wound Healing Guidelines and Guidance (Continued)

Stages of healing for surgical wounds of primary intention (approximated incisions):

A. **Fully granulating/healing:** Incision is well approximated with complete epithelialization of incision; no signs or symptoms of infection; healing ridge is well defined.

B. **Early/partial granulation:** Incision is well approximated but not completely epithelialized; no signs or symptoms of infection; healing ridge is palpable but poorly defined.

C. **Non-healing:** Incisional separation *OR* Incisional necrosis *OR* no palpable healing ridge

Stages of healing for surgical wounds by secondary intention (healing of dehisced wounds by granulation, contraction, and epithelialization)

A. **Fully granulating:** Wound bed is filled with granulation tissue to the level of the surrounding skin or new epithelium; no dead space; no signs of infection; wound edges are open.

B. **Early/Partial granulation:** More than 25% of the wound bed is covered with granulation tissue; there is minimal avascular tissue (>25% of the wound bed is covered with avascular tissue); may have dead space; no signs of infection; wound edges are open.

C. **Non-healing:** Wound with more than 25% avascular tissue *OR* signs of infection *OR* clean but non-granulation wound bed *OR* closed/hyperkeratotic wound edges *OR* persistent failure to improve despite comprehensive appropriate wound management.

Glossary

Avascular: Lacking in blood supply; dead, devitalized, necrotic, non-viable. Slough and eschar

Clean wound: Wound free of devitalized tissue, purulent drainage, foreign material or debris

Closed wound: Top layers of epidermis have rolled down to cover wound

Dead space: A defect or cavity

Dehisced/dehiscence: Separation of surgical incision; loss of approximation of wound edges

Edges: Lower edge of epidermis, including basement membrane, so that epithelial cells cannot migrate from wound edges, also described as *epibole*. Presents clinically as sealed edge of mature epithelium; may be hard/thickened; may be discolored (yellow, gray, or white)

Epidermis: Outermost layer of the skin

Epithelialization: Regeneration of epidermis across a wound surface

Eschar: Black or brown necrotic, devitalized tissue; tissue that can be firmly or loosely adherent, hard, soft, or soggy

Full thickness: Tissue damage involving total loss of epidermis and dermis and extending into the subcutaneous tissue and possibly into the muscle or bone

Granulation tissue: The pink/red, moist tissue composed of new blood vessels, connective tissue, fibroblasts, and inflammatory cells that fill an open wound when it starts to heal; typically appears deep pink or red with an irregular "berry-like" surface

Healing: A dynamic process involving synthesis of new tissue for repair of skin and soft tissue defects

Healing ridge: Palpatory finding indicative of new collagen synthesis. Palpation reveals induration beneath the skin that extends to approximately 1cm on each side of the wound. This becomes evident between 5 and 9 days after wounding; typically persists until about 15 days post wounding; this is an expected positive sign

Hyperkeratosis: Hard, white/gray tissue surrounding the wound

Infection: The presence of bacteria or other microorganisms in sufficient quantity to damage tissue or impair healing. Wounds can be classified as infected when the wound tissue contains 100,000 or greater microorganisms per gram of tissue. Typical signs and symptoms of infection include purulent exudate, odor, erythema, warmth, tenderness, edema, pain, fever, and an elevated white cell count. However, clinical signs of infection may not be present, especially in the immunocompromised patient or the patient with poor tissue perfusion.

Necrotic tissue: Same as avascular

Non-granulating: Absence of granulation tissue; wound surface appears smooth as opposed to granular (for example, in a wound that is clean but non-granulating, the wound surface appears smooth and red as opposed to "berry-like")

Partial thickness: Confined to skin layers; damage does not penetrate below the skin dermis and may be limited to the dermal layers only

Sinus tract: Course or path of tissue destruction occurring in any direction from the surface or edge of the wound; results in dead space with potential for abscess formation; also called "tunneling" (can be distinguished from undermining by the fact that the sinus tract involves a small portion of the wound edge whereas undermining involves a significant portion of the wound edge).

Slough: Soft moist avascular (devitalized) tissue; may be white, yellow, tan, or green; may be loose or firmly adherent

Tunneling: See sinus tract

Undermining: Area of tissue destruction extending under intact skin along the periphery of the wound; commonly seen in shear injuries; can be distinguished from sinus tract by the fact that undermining involves a significant portion of the wound edge, whereas sinus tract involves only a small portion of the wound edge.

2. Consistently following policies and procedures can help staff fully adopt and understand the special needs of older adult patients. Staff training and education, coupled with ongoing monitoring and tracking of adherence to these policies, should be a part of any overall strategy.

Buccellato offers advice on the importance of enforcing policies and procedures. "It is worthwhile to note that the enforcement of policies and procedures will be more effective if the staff/stakeholders of the processes, in the policy, are included as the policy is being developed or at least are able to review the policy before it is implemented," Buccellato notes. "At this time, any new processes that may have a negative impact on other current processes can be identified and 'fixed.' Eliminating these elements of review can make the difference between success and failure of a new policy," states Buccellato.

To help ensure and encourage staff adherence to any new or revised policy and procedure, consider the following tips:

Educate and Orient. Make sure you factor in plenty of opportunities to orient staff to the new policies and procedures, particularly if the revisions or new material signals a significantly new process. It is important to keep in mind a variety of approaches to education as well; not all staff members learn the same way, and not all will retain information in the same manner. It can also be particularly helpful to provide background information and education on why these changes are taking place. Understanding the importance of why a change has to take place can often help staff embrace making that change.

Report on success and progress along the way. If one organization has made a change to its falls risk assessment procedure to help reduce the number of patient falls, for example, and begins to track progress based on implementing the new policy and procedure, it should report progress to staff. Many of these changes require commitment and consistent effort on the part of staff, and making those changes should be encouraged and celebrated along the way.

Let these efforts become part of the culture of safety. No one process or system that ensures patient safety should be regarded as "more important" than anything else. As staff begin to see all elements of ensuring patient safety as important aspects of their jobs, it becomes more "business as usual" and not just another requirement of the job.

Make sure efforts are sustained. Don't just make changes, make sure they are sustainable. Carefully introduce and implement changes that staff can embrace and work toward. One helpful way to approach this is to ensure you have staff buy-in to the process. This can be achieved by having key staff members—especially frontline staff—involved in assessing and making changes to the policy and procedure and in providing feedback on how progress is being made.

Communication Between Shift Changes

An important aspect of communication between staff is what happens at shift change in the hospital or long term care setting. This is one of those important events in the care of a patient where staff communicate key information to each other—the effective shift change means that there is little to no disruption to the care experience of the patient, and crucial information is communicated effectively to the next staff member. This transition can be particularly important to an older adult patient, who may feel vulnerable, anxious, or unsure with a new staff member. Managing that shift change with the patient in mind can help ensure patient safety and benefit staff. Consider the following suggestions when looking at how well your staff manages shift changes:

Rethink where you conduct shift changes. Some hospitals have begun doing shift changes at the bedside. This can take away the opportunity for a more focused discussion among staff of a unit at shift change time, but it can allow for a face-to-face introduction by the outgoing staff of the incoming staff to the patient and family. It can also help staff reiterate key patient care issues and reinforce crucial patient education in the patient's presence. This could also reinforce a supportive interpersonal communication between staff and patients.

Make sure the crucial issues are consistently shared. If an older adult patient is determined to be at high risk for falls or had a pressure ulcer, for example, ensure there is a process to clearly identify these issues at shift change times.

Training and Orientation of New Staff Members

With the population seeing an increase in the proportion of its older adult–aged members, health care organizations are facing an increase in the number of older adult patients they care for. This rise is not being met with adequate numbers of health care workers with specific training in caring for older adult patients.[5] It may not always be practical to recruit staff with particular training in older adult care, so organizations need to ensure that they have adequately planned for the training and orientation of new staff to know how to care for older adult patients.

When planning their orientation and training for new staff in relation to older adult patients, organizations should consider the following special areas of concern that can face older adult patients:

- Skin assessment, wound care, and pressure ulcers
- Falls risk assessment, falls prevention
- Medication reconciliation and safety
- Memory and mental status
- Nutrition and hydration
- Abuse and neglect
- Patient and family interaction and education

Organizations can approach training and orientation in different ways. Consider the following tips when planning for training and orientation:

Vary the approach. Don't provide only one style of training or orientation—ensure that the knowledge is provided in different styles that help as many staff members understand the communication strategies as possible.

Involve leadership. Leadership can have a big impact on helping staff understand and appreciate a culture of safety, so ensure they are part of any orientation process and any significant training sessions.

Initial Communication

The initial contact that an older adult patient has with an organization is important to that care experience. When done well, the assessment, care planning, and communication process with an older adult patient can lay an important foundation for the ongoing safe care of that patient. The following section discusses common challenges for organizations with initial communication in relation to older adult patients: assessment, patient-provider communication, medication reconciliation, handoff communication, inter- and intradisciplinary communication, and external communication.

Assessment of Older Adult Patients

For all patients, an assessment is an essential means by which a health care organization can begin to plan for care. This is often a robust approach that requires that the organization have an effective process prepared to assess patients and that patients be engaged to provide comprehensive information. In the case of an older adult patient, additional steps should be in place to gauge if the patient is at risk for such things as falls, pressure ulcers, memory loss, nutrition, and pain. Table 1-1, pages 9–10, describes the kinds of assessment tools that can be used in relation to older adult assessment.

A multitude of assessment tools is available for organizations to use, and the literature has indicated that this diversity makes knowing which tool to use problematic.[6] One approach to determining the best way to assess older adult patients might be to adopt a tool that has been studied in the literature and adapt, as appropriate, to the needs of your organization. A key element to integrate into any attempt to introduce a new or revised assessment approach is adequate training and monitoring of the tool's success. When adopting any assessment, it should be suitable for your type of health care setting, be manageable for staff to use, and help ensure that any high risks are identified and

Table 1-1. Older Adult Patient Assessment Tools

Type of Assessment	Description	Examples of Tools
Falls Risk Assessment	These assessments allow an organization to ascertain what level of risk a patient may have for falls while under the care of a health care organization.	One challenge in the area of falls risk assessment is that although many tools are available, research is noting that some of these tools have not been tested for reliability or validity.[7] The Minnesota Falls Prevention Initiative (http://www.mnfallsprevention.org/professional/assessmenttools.html) offers a few commonly used assessment tools to consider: ■ *Taking Action to Prevent Falls:* This assessment tool, from Fall Prevention Center of Excellence (http://www.stopfalls.org), can be used for assessment in the home. ■ *Check For Safety:* The Centers for Disease Control and Prevention (CDC) has designed a checklist, *A Home Fall Prevention Checklist for Older Adults*, for home safety assessment (http://www.cdc.gov/ncipc/pub-res/toolkit/Falls_ToolKit/Offset/English/booklet_Eng_offset.pdf). ■ *STRATIFY:* A tool that identifies risk factors and creates a risk profile score. Used to identify clinical fall risk factors in the elderly and to predict chance of falling.[8] ■ *Morse Fall Scale:* Recommended for inpatient settings, such as hospitals and long term care settings.[9] ■ *Hendrich Fall Risk Assessment:* Recommended by the National Center for Patient Safety for inpatients. Used in some long term care settings. *See* Chapter 5 for more examples of these assessment tools, among others.
Nutritional Screening Tools	Nutrition is often a risk factor for older adult patients. Having an effective assessment of a patient's nutritional status can help a health care organization care effectively for patients and prevent any risk that could come from poor nutritional status.	The following is an example of a nutritional status tool: ■ *DETERMINE:* A tool from the American Academy of Family Physicians, the National Council on the Aging, and others as part of the Nutrition Screening Initiative. This tool can be used to assess risk for poor nutritional status or malnutrition (http://www.aafp.org).

continued

Table 1-1. Older Adult Patient Assessment Tools (Continued)

Type of Assessment	Description	Examples of Tools
Pressure Ulcer Risk Assessment	Although it is rare that a decubitis ulcer, or a pressure ulcer, will be a direct cause of the death of a patient, it is often linked to a sequence of negative outcomes for an older adult patient that can lead toward decline. Assessing and monitoring an older adult patient for pressure ulcer risk is essential for his or her continued patient safety.	Although there are not as many different assessment tools or guidelines for assessing pressure ulcer risk as there are with falls risk, quite a few have been developed. The following represent a few commonly used tools: ■ *Pressure Ulcer Prevention Points:* A concise document brought by the National Pressure Ulcer Advisory Panel (NPUAP) that lists the key risk points to consider in relation to the risk of developing pressure ulcers (http://www.npuap.org/PU_Prev_Points.pdf). ■ *The Norton Scale:* A rating scale for risk factors used for inpatients; the lower the score, the higher the risk factors (http://www.ncbi.nlm.nih.gov/books/bv.fcgi?rid=hstat2.table.4948). ■ *The Braden Scale for Predicting Pressure Sore Risk:* The Braden Scale is a scoring tool that allows organizations to rate a patient's risk for developing pressure ulcers (http://www.bradenscale.com/bradenscale.htm). ■ *The Waterlow Scale:* The Waterlow Scale predicts risk for pressure ulcer development (http://www.judy-waterlow.co.uk/waterlow_score.htm). *See* Chapter 8 for more information on pressure ulcers and examples of assessment tools.
Pain Assessment Tools	Pain is a predominant concern for older adult patients and should be assessed correctly.	Pain is a serious issue for any patient, but is a particular concern for older adult patients. Consider using the following pain assessment tools: ■ Visual analog scales ■ Numeric pain intensity scale ■ Simple descriptive pain intensity scale ■ Graphic rating scale ■ Verbal rating scale ■ Pain faces scale ■ Numeric pain intensity and pain distress scales ■ Brief pain inventory

managed in a timely manner. Sidebar 1-1, page 12, explores the concept of assessment in further detail.

In addition, organizations may have to consider what other types of assessments may be required of them by state, federal, or other governing agencies. For example, home care agencies may be required to adhere to OASIS by CMS, or a long term care organization may be required to adhere to minimum data set (MDS) assessment criteria.

Medication Reconciliation

Medication has long been considered an area with significant patient safety concerns. Medication errors can lead to unwanted adverse events. Organizations are being asked by federal and state regulating bodies and by such accrediting agencies as The Joint Commission to carefully manage their medication management systems to reduce sentinel events. Although medication safety for older adult patients is handled in greater detail in Chapter 3, the following comments highlight some of the crucial communication aspects to keep in mind when communicating with older adult patients on medications and, in particular, regarding medication reconciliation.

Polypharmacy

The issue of polypharmacy, or the use of multiple medications by patients, is particularly pressing for older adult patients who tend to be impacted by polypharmacy far more than younger patients. As a result, the need for effective medication reconciliation is an essential aspect of any communication relationship with an older adult patient, particularly at important times of transition, such as admission or discharge. Organizations need to ensure that patients' use of medications is well documented and assessed to prevent any unintended adverse interactions or impact to the patient.

Medication reconciliation is the process by which an organization creates a list or documents the medication that a patient is on when admitted to an organization and during the process of receiving care, treatment, and services. The fact that the lack of proper medication reconciliation can lead to adverse events has caused The Joint Commission to require that accredited health care organizations comply with a National Patient Safety Goal that states that a process has to exist for comparing the patient's current medications with those ordered for the patient while under the care of the organization. For older adult patients who may be taking more than the average number of medications, it is essential for organizations to carefully track and document what is being used; in addition, ensuring that medication lists are communicated to other organizations when that patient is discharged is essential.

Older adult patients should be worked with to clearly communicate which medications they are taking, including nonprescription medications. Patient education and ongoing communication about medication use and interactions are good ways to help patients understand the importance of medication safety. The patient must understand what medications he or she needs to take on discharge. This topic is discussed in greater depth in Chapter 3.

Communicating Patients' Needs: Handoff Communication and Discharge

Handoff Communication

Another important area where communication plans play a crucial role in preventing adverse events is in relation to handoff communication. Patients will often navigate many components of a health care organization, even if they are being moved between departments. Any time a patient receives additional care or is moved into another aspect of his or her care experience determines how the organization communicates key elements of handoffs. Handoffs are particularly important in the following ways:

- *Inter- and intradisciplinary communication.* It is crucial that an organization have well-designed processes in place to enable staff to effectively communicate with each other. Many handoffs take place within an institution, especially at a hospital, and well-communicated handoffs can have an important impact on patient safety. The patient's record can also include a lot of crucial information that should be communicated across disciplines.
- *Outside the department.* If a patient is moving through different departments of an institution—going, for example, from the gastrointerology lab to radiology—or receiving care from different departments—from nutrition to respiratory therapy—handoff communications are crucial.
- *Outside the organization.* It is important to maintain effective lines of communication between organizations,

Sidebar 1-1. Assessment: Collecting Patient Information

What are some steps in the assessment process?

Assessment includes such aspects as collecting, recording, analyzing, and interpreting data/information. Methods of data/information collection can include:

- Screening
- Assessment
- Reassessment
- Interviewing
- Examination and testing

Who contributes data/information to the assessment process?

Data/information can be gathered from the following:

- Patient
- Primary care team
- Multidisciplinary team members
- Family members, friends and/or caregiver
- Previous medical records, if available

Assessment tools can help determine risk, but they are most effective when used together with clinical judgment.

Why does assessment matter?

Assessment identifies an area, or areas, of need. It can help health care providers identify actual and/or potential problems or issues. It forms the basis for care planning and treatment. Re-assessment in the process of evaluation identifies the success or failure of interventions that have been implemented and identifies needs that have not been addressed.[10]

especially if an older adult patient has been receiving care from another organization. This is particularly important in the case of a long term care resident, for example, who may have been admitted to the hospital for treatment or a procedure. If an adverse event takes place, such as the development of a pressure ulcer or a patient fall, this should be communicated to the outside organization. The patient's history of risks, such as a history of pressure ulcers or patient falls, should be communicated between organizations so the receiving organization can appropriately plan for any high risks.

Discharge Instructions

Discharge is often a crucial point in a patient's care experience. He or she may be leaving the hospital with multiple medical problems that could require he or she be admitted into home care, or he or she could be going from a hospital into a long term care setting. At these times, the patient and family may feel additional stress, not being sure how the next stage in treatment and care will go or knowing that they have to take on additional responsibilities for care. It could also be a transitional time in that patient's life, when he or she entered the acute care setting feeling healthy and fully functional and may be going home with far more limitations than before.

Because discharge is often a time in care when an organization must ensure that the patient and family understand instructions for postdischarge care and prepare for a new stage in the care process, clear communication is essential. If a patient is being discharged from a hospital into home care, for example, the hospital must ensure that the home care agency receives ample information about the incoming patient. The more streamlined and organized this process is, the lesser chance there is for an adverse event or for the patient to experience any worsening of his or her condition. The hospital also has to communicate to the home care agency any high-risk determinations made about the patient while in the hospital, such as if the patient was deemed to be at high risk for falls or developed a pressure ulcer. Medication reconciliation is also a crucial aspect of the discharge process. The discharging institution should provide a list of all medications used for the patient as well as providing any necessary education and demonstrations on using medications or treatments. It's a good idea to not only provide this kind of education at the time of discharge but also to prepare the family and patient for the information by sharing with them sooner as well. Thus, the education provided at the time of discharge can be a way to verify that the family and patient understand their postdischarge instructions (and can even demonstrate that understanding) and have an opportunity to ask any questions if they are unsure. Discharging organizations should also consider integrating a "follow-up" process by which they can phone the patient and/or family following discharge to see if any questions or concerns may have come up since being discharged.

Patients and Families

Probably one of the most important aspects of communication, particularly as a patient safety strategy, is the communication between care providers and patients and families. Clear communication and education between providers and patients can help close the loop on important aspects of delivering care and in engaging patients in being actively involved in their own patient safety. This kind of active involvement has been shown to help increase patient safety and also increase a patient's satisfaction with his or her care.

It was not always customary or considered acceptable for patients to have such an active involvement in their own care, however. Until recent years, it was customary for the provider-patient relationship to be a one-way communication: from the provider to the patient. The patient would often passively receive instruction and just be expected to understand and follow the instructions, and the provider retained responsibility for caring for the patient and ensuring his or her safety. It was the culture not to question the doctor, for example, or to query a health care worker about any instructions received. This more common "patient culture" in health care was prevalent in recent decades and is still having an impact on whether patients will feel free to engage in open dialogue with health care providers.

Older adult patients may be more accustomed to the more traditional style of health care and as a result may be less willing to engage in an open dialogue with their health care providers about any of their patient safety concerns. This makes it even more important that health care organizations refine and hone their ability to communicate effectively with older adult patients and their families. Considering the complexity of risks and health care conditions that an older adult patient may carry with him or her into a health care organization, empowering older adult patients to be engaged in their own care is especially important to ensuring their patient safety.

Communicating Effectively with Patients and Family Members

Communication is an essential factor for determining patient satisfaction with their care.[11] Although an older adult patient may not be used to expressing a desire for interpersonal communication in a health care setting, it is extremely important to encourage that level of communication. It not only helps provide for a more satisfying care experience for the older adult patient but can also make an important difference in preventing adverse events. Some qualities of effective communication include ongoing clear lines of contact between patients and providers, good listening skills, empathy and social interaction, and the use of a variety of communication techniques.

Communication not only is important when a patient is initially admitted to an organization but is a crucial part of an ongoing relationship. Undergoing medical care can be a stressful experience for an older adult patient, particularly as he or she may be facing a number of conditions and progressively complicated health problems. This section explores some important aspects of communication between providers and older adult patients and family members: listening, training staff on communication skills, involving families in patient care, communication under special circumstances, and the use of a variety of communication approaches.

Listening: The Heart of Communication

For many older adult patients, knowing they are being listened to can be particularly important in establishing a good relationship with their health care providers. In studies conducted in long term care settings, it has been determined that being listened to is fundamental to a resident's quality of life.[2] In fact, listening has long been seen as an essential part of nursing.[2] When a patient feels he or she is being genuinely listened to, it helps establish the provider-patient relationship, which can help prevent patients from being unwilling or unsure about sharing any concerns about their care.

However, not all staff have had an opportunity to develop listening skills, particularly in a health care environment. In the midst of a busy work environment with a great deal of care-related tasks to perform, it can be hard to find a way to balance that with taking the time to listen and connect with a patient. Training sessions with staff can help encourage an atmosphere where listening is nurtured and help them learn important listening skills in the process. Consider the empathy-building exercise on page 14 as a way for staff to reflect on what being listened to might mean to them, which can help them relate to what it might mean for a patient. This exercise can be done in small groups.

These kinds of exercises can help staff pause in their busy work schedules to reflect on what the care experience

Listening Empathy Exercise[2]

Have staff reflect on the meaning of being listened to.

- Share an anecdote of a time when you felt listened to.
- What does it mean to you to be listened to?
- What does it feel like when you know you're being listened to?

Staff should take time to describe the patterns of relating, which are connected to being listened to.

- What are your relationships like when you are being listened to?
- How does being listened to change those relationships?

Staff should describe what they hope for when they are being listened to.

- If you were the patient in this health care organization, what would be important to you, as far as being listened to?
- What helps you when it comes to being listened to?
- What do you hope for when it comes to being listened to?

might mean to patients, particularly while they and their family are in the midst of a stressful, anxiety-ridden experience. It can take time to develop effective listening skills, but ongoing, supportive training can help staff adopt them into their everyday activities. In fact, another helpful way for staff to work on their listening skills is through the process of their care activities. When a staff member conducts an assessment, he or she can take that opportunity to engage the older adult patient in discussion and focus on listening to the patient.

A few important qualities of listening include the following:

- *Eye contact.* Stopping other activities and focusing on the speaker can go a long way toward reassuring him or her that you are really listening.
- *Making time.* Take time to let patients articulate their response. Do not rush them or cut them off.
- *Reflecting.* Reassure the person speaking that you are listening by reflecting on what you are hearing. For example, "So as I understand it, you felt confused when we were educating you on this new prescription, and you're worried that you will make a mistake?"
- *Encouragement.* Sometimes a patient wants to share but may be hesitant. Using encouraging statements such as "Please tell me more" or "Can you share more about that?" can help the patient feel supported and listened to.
- *Take your time.* Do not rush any conversations with an older adult patient.

Elderspeak: A Common Pitfall in Communicating with Older Adult Patients

Sometimes an unexpected pitfall in communicating with older adult patients is the use of what is called "elderspeak," a kind of speech that is similar to "baby talk."[3] Staff often do this unintentionally, but it can communicate a lack of respect, imply incompetence, and appear patronizing to the listener. Elderspeak is described as often taking place between younger staff and older adult patients and seems more prevalent in settings where older adult patients are primarily cared for, such as a long term care setting. Qualities of elderspeak are characterized as the use of diminutives ("honey," "good girl"), inappropriate plural pronoun use ("Are *we* going to take *our* medicine today?"), tag questions ("You would rather have the sweet corn, *wouldn't you*?"), and slow, loud speech. Unfortunately, elderspeak may have negative impacts on a patient's self-esteem, could trigger depression, and could withdraw an older adult patient from social interaction.[12]

Research has found that there are a variety of ways staff can communicate with older adult patients. Consider the following examples of how a staff member might communicate to a resident of a long term care facility who appears disoriented and is wandering into the wrong room:

- **Overly nurturing talk:** Highly caring, not controlling, inappropriately intimate (for example, "Where do you think you're going, sweetie? That's not your room, honey.")
- **Directive talk:** Highly controlling, no recognition of listener's autonomy, little caring (for example, "That's not your room. You can't be there, residents aren't supposed to go into those rooms.")
- **Affirming talk:** Balanced care and control (for example, "Mr. Ramirez, it looks like you are lost. Are you having trouble finding your room? May I show you back to your room?")[3]

Although all three approaches respond to the patient and may correct his or her confusion, the "affirming talk" approach allows the staff member to remain caring and compassionate, employ a respectful tone, and actively engage the patient in acting to help resolve the problem.

Training staff to be aware of how they communicate and adjust their tone, if appropriate, could reduce the incidence of elderspeak. Consider the following strategies when working with staff to be aware of elderspeak and avoid using it:

Strategy

Survey patients to see what their experiences have been. Ask patients if they feel that communication is effective. If there is an overall perception of elderspeak, share that with your staff. If staff learn that patients feel the communication is not responsive to their needs, it can often be easier for staff to be open to making a change.

Strategy

Engage all staff in exercises to think about what they say and to whom. Do an exercise with staff where they write down what they say during a visit with a patient. Ask them to anonymously document what they hear colleagues saying to patients. Share those in a group and decide what, if any, statements seem to employ elderspeak.

Strategy

Brainstorm alternative ways to communicate with a patient. Invite staff, in a training session, to come up with alternative ways to communicate that do not employ elderspeak:

Elderspeak: "Let's take that medicine, sweetie."
Alternative: "Here is your medicine, Mrs. Jones."
Elderspeak: "Shall we put our socks on?"
Alternative: "Are you ready to put your socks on?"
Elderspeak: "You would prefer to eat the pudding, wouldn't you?"
Alternative: "Would you like to have the pudding?"

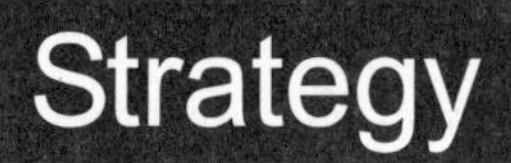

Encourage staff to practice using "affirming" talk. Prepare typical scenarios that may take place in your health care organization and ask staff to come up with and practice ways of using an affirming tone to respond to a patient.

Family and Older Adult Patients: Discussing Care and Treatment and Providing Patient and Family Education

For many older adult patients, family involvement in their care is often a given. For health care providers, this can be an important benefit to ensuring the well being and safety of the older adult patient. Consider the following ways to involve patients and families in patient education and discussing their care and treatment:

Encourage the patient to bring a companion on visits or have a companion or family member with him or her when receiving important instructions. Although this may not be desirable for all patients or suitable in every circumstance, an older adult patient may benefit from having a trusted companion accompanying him or her on doctors' visits or when receiving important information or instructions.

Reinforce education by discussing it with both the patient and the family throughout the care process, not just right before discharge. Being under medical care—especially in an acute care setting—can be an overwhelming and intimidating experience. Ensure that the patient and family understand what they should expect during care and after discharge by giving plenty of opportunities to discuss it. Waiting until right before a patient is discharged can make things confusing for the patient and family and could mean that key pieces of information are lost.

Restore the reciprocity of care for patients coming into long term care settings by encouraging story sharing. It can take a while for a resident to become accustomed to being in a long term care facility. He or she is transitioning from the more common adult experience of the "give and take" of caring into a situation where he or she is being cared for. This can be a significant transition for both the older adult patient and the family. One effective intervention to help with the adjustment is "story sharing." Story sharing is a "two-way, ongoing process of enriching relationships that permits access to personal meanings, beliefs, and values and is accessible to all levels of caregivers."[13] This storytelling involves both the staff member and the patient taking turns sharing stories with each other. This can build important bonds of trust, a sharing of commonalities, and connection between staff and patients, and it can be readily applied in the long term care or home care settings, for example.

Use a variety of communication techniques. Consider e-mail bulletins or other electronic communication to provide ongoing patient and family education. In the case of long term care settings, promote the use of videophones or other voice-over communication techniques to keep patients and their family connected.

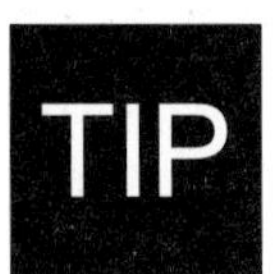

Encourage collaborative participation for family members. Although this may not be suitable in some acute care setting situations, it can be helpful for family members to be involved in multidisciplinary care planning for older adult patients, particularly in a long term care setting.[14] The role of a family member in a collaborative multidisciplinary team could be helpful to allow them to ask questions, share important concerns about problems for the patient, and raise any other relevant issues that may require consideration in making a care plan.[14]

Handling Special Communication Situations

In some situations, an older adult patient may have special concerns, which could require a particular response from the health care organization. These include the following:

Communicating with patients and families with language and cultural barriers: Organizations should be sure to consider the different communications issues or concerns that could arise with patients and families who have cultural or language barriers. For example, it may feel inappropriate for a female patient of a particular culture or religious background to receive personal care assistance from a male staff member. Organizations should work closely with patients to learn what, if any, particular concerns or limitations may exist for them. In addition, translation services should be available to patients and their families.

Communicating regarding abuse or neglect: It can be particularly challenging for an organization to know how to cope with incidences of abuse or neglect, particularly when it impacts a vulnerable older adult patient. Organizations should put in place effective assessment processes to prevent the incidence of abuse or neglect and also work to communicate with patients and families about how to spot cases of abuse and neglect. For example, a home care agency can work with patients and families to educate them on how to spot and avoid cases of self-neglect on the part of the older adult patient. *See* Chapter 8 for more information on assessing for and dealing with abuse and neglect.

Depression or suicide risk: The ways that older adult patients deal with and approach depression and suicide are quite different from younger patients. Organizations need to ensure that they are regularly assessing and discussing danger signs with patients and families.

Cognitive issues: Older adult patients face a number of challenges in communication, including hearing problems, mental issues, mood disorders, or cognitive disorders. Patients with such limitations may require a special communication approach. Patients with hearing or vision impairment should be accommodated with added visual or hearing aids to help them communicate or understand. In the case of older adult patients with dementia, for example, staff may need to use such techniques as exploring (searching for information about a patient) or clarifying (attempting to ensure that the staff member understands the patient).[15] Consider Sidebar 1-2 for a list of suggested techniques to use with cognitively impaired patients.

Sidebar 1-2. Taxonomy of Nurse Interactions with Residents Who Have Dementia

Clarifying: Attempting to ensure that the nurse understood the resident (for example, repeating, restating, asking questions to understand residents' statements, and acknowledging inability to understand resident)

Exploring: Searching for information (usually with a question) about the individual resident and helping him or her articulate a personal experience or view of the topic (for example, asking about environment, self [that is, family, friends, and personal history], perceptions, or preferences)

Moderating: Initiating and maintaining the general conversation (for example, introducing topics, maintaining flow, expanding topic with statement, steering back to topic, making statements that imply or give direction, answering questions, drawing on knowledge of resident, shutting down "hot topics," finishing off/pulling together)

Validating: Recognizing expressed or inferred feelings (verbal or nonverbal) (for example, supporting; reassuring; making a positive comment, such as well done; suggesting a feeling)

Rescuing: Suggesting relevance for specific, isolated, or unconnected statements (for example, suggesting answers, options, solutions; picking up on phrases and making a connection; providing context for a comment; offering assistance; providing a word or phrase; correcting residents' understanding)

Discourse Markers: Using strategies that fit with social/generational expectations (for example, social conventions, such as "thank you"; acknowledging comments, such as "OK" or "Uh-huh"; orientating/focusing; checking audibility of conversations; explaining own actions)

Connecting: Establishing a link between the group leaders and resident, between the topic and the resident, or between residents (for example, using personal information about self, drawing upon knowledge of resident, identifying common experiences)

Assisting: Asking about and physically supporting resident comfort (for example, physical comfort, place in the group)

Source: *Perry J., et al.: Communication in dementia: Improving the odds.* J Gerontol Nurs, *31(4):43–52 Apr. 2005.*

Conclusion

At the core of any effective relationship between health care provider and patient is communication. Good communication helps ensure effective assessment, care planning, treatment, transitions in care and discharge, and patient and family education. In fact, the entire continuum of care is strengthened by consistent and well-functioning streams of communication. Considering the complexity of health care concerns and potential risks that older adult patients face, the need for good communication is particularly pressing for health care organizations to consider. The next chapter, Chapter 2, considers another important area for organizations to consider in ensuring older adult patient safety: the physical environment of health care.

References

1. "Nonprofit Cites 10 Common Errors Medical Professionals Make When Communicating with Their Patients." http://www.reuters.com/article/pressRelease/idUS218365+13-Aug-2008+MW20080813 (accessed Feb. 19, 2009).
2. Jonas-Simpson et al.: The experience of being listened to. *J Gerontol Nurs,* 32(1):46–53 Jan. 2006.
3. Williams K., et al.: Enhancing communication with older adults: Overcoming elderspeak. *J Gerontol Nurs,* 30(10):17–25 Oct. 2004.
4. Williams K.N., Ilten T.B.: meeting communication needs: Topics

of talk in the nursing home. *J Psychosoc Nurs Ment Health Serv* 43(7):38–45 Jul. 2005.

5. Lewis R.C.: Medical schools prepare for "silver tsunami." http://www.reuters.com/article/latestCrisis/idUSN28499322 (accessed Feb. 19, 2009).
6. Toofany S.: Tools to care. *Nursing Older People* 19(10): 13–5, Dec. 2007.
7. Myers H.: Hospital fall risk assessment tools: a critique of the literature. *Int J Nurs Pract* 9(4):223–235, 2003.
8. Oliver D., et al.: Development and evaluation of evidence based risk assessment tool (STRATIFY) to predict which elderly inpatients will fall: Case-control and cohort studies. http://www.bmj.com/cgi/content/full/315/7115/1049 (accessed Feb. 19, 2009).
9. Morse J.M., Morse R.M., Tylko S.J.: Development of a scale to identify the fall-prone patient. *Can J Aging* 8(4):366–367, 1989.
10. Armstrong J., Mitchell E.: Comprehensive nursing assessment in the care of older people. *Nurs Older People* 20(1):36–40, Feb. 2008.
11. Grau L., Chandler B., Saunders C.: Nursing home residents' perceptions of the quality of their care. *J Psychosoc Nurs Ment Health Serv* 33(5):34–41, 1995.
12. Kemper S., Harden T.: Experimentally disentangling what's beneficial about elderspeak from what's not. *Psychol and Aging* 14(1):55–73, 1999.
13. Heliker D.: Story sharing. *J Psychosoc Nurs Ment Health Serv* 45(7):20–23, Jul. 2007.
14. Dijkstra A.: Family participation. *J Gerontol Nurs* pp. 22–30, Apr. 2007.
15. Perry J., et al.: Nurse-patient communication in dementia. *J Gerontol Nurs* p. 46, Apr. 2005.

Chapter 2

Improving the Physical Environment for Older Adults

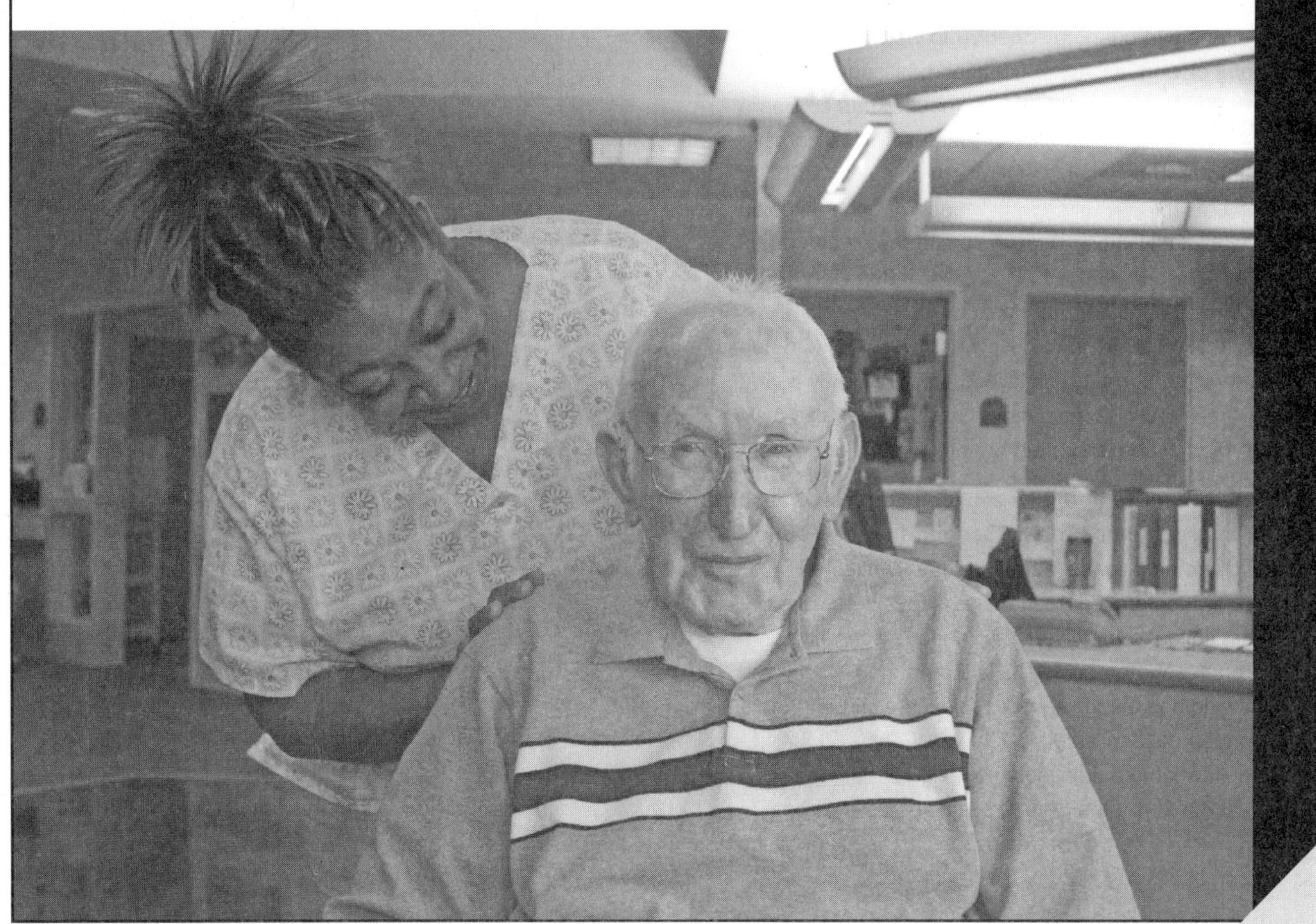

Just as communication is paramount in older adult patients' safety, the physical environment plays a prominent role as well. The health care industry is facing caring for an aging population that not only is increasingly impacting the ability of health care organizations to cope with their medical needs but also may not be well prepared for the unique environmental challenges that older adult patients face. They may have a high risk for falls and pressure ulcers, be physically more fragile and vulnerable, be on multiple medications that could disorient them, or could have cognitive disorders that could require extra environmental interventions to reduce their risk of harm.

Although this book's focus is primarily on the urgency of ensuring that an organization's environment is safe for older adult patients, a word should be said about the growing movement and understanding that the environment itself can also be therapeutic, which can go a long way toward helping patients be safe and well.[1] In fact, some studies have found that a combination of environmental, behavioral, and pharmacological approaches can be effective in improving the health, clinical outcomes, safety, and quality of life of Alzheimer's patients in special care units.[2]

Although an organization should keep safety as a paramount concern in its design, it can also keep in mind that a nurturing environment that helps empower and support a patient can be important to his or her well being and safety as well. In fact, some studies have found that unconventional long term care settings, such as the Green House®, a living model for long term care that is designed as a small living community for residents and staff, are having a positive impact on the well being and satisfaction of residents. Concepts such as the Green House model require differences in reconsidering such elements of an organization as facility size, interior design, staffing patterns, and methods of delivering care, treatment, and services.[3–5]

Solid care, systems, and processes to provide such things as good communication and assessment are important aspects of helping reduce the incidence of older adult patient adverse events. In addition, the environment itself can play an important role in ensuring that patients remain safe. This chapter explores how organizations should look at their environment or their patients' interaction with their own environment to ensure they reduce the risk of an adverse event and also discuss any particular geriatric patient-related issues in relation to emergency management. When it comes to the environment of care (EC), also known as the physical environment, health care organizations can differ quite a bit from each other, such as in the case of EC issues for a home care agency as compared to those in a hospital. Therefore, although some aspects of this chapter may apply universally across settings, some elements may only apply to specific settings.

The Physical Environment and Older Adult Patients

Is your organization prepared to provide a safe environment for older adult patients? Have you built in measures that help prevent falls? What provisions do you have in place in the event of a wandering patient? How are you assessing risks in the home for home care patients? How do you educate patients and families about preparing their environment—or being mindful of their environment—to prevent any adverse events?

"The environment is an important issue for organizations to keep in mind when considering safety of geriatric patients," says Elaine Buccellato, B.S.N., M.S., Joint Commission surveyor in long term care and hospital settings. "An organization should be flexible and creative in looking at ways to ensure the safety of their geriatric patients. Included in this approach, the organization needs to promote independent functioning of geriatric patients by assuring that the physical environment and processes of care do not impede functional independence." Buccellato states that key items may allay the effects of functional decline and make the physical environment safer for the older adult patient:

1. The use of adjustable "hi-low" beds
2. Adaptive equipment
3. Handrails
4. Uncluttered rooms and hallways
5. Elevated toilet seats
6. Call bells within patient's reach

Buccellato also points to a benefit that a Joint Commission survey can bring to hospitals. "Now that we have *Life Safety Code*®* specialists on surveys, they will be

* Life Safety Code® *is a registered trademark of the National Fire Protection Association, Quincy, MA.*

looking at safety issues throughout, including those faced by geriatric patients."

Risk Factors for the Older Adult Population

Older adult patients face a lot of risks in the environment of a health care organization: everything from poorly functioning medical equipment to design elements that could negatively impact a patient's safety. The following are some of the most common risk factors faced by older adult patients in the environment:

- *Patient falls.* Falls not only are the most prevalent adverse event in hospitals but also happen in other health care settings.[2] Putting safeguards into the environment, coupled with education and assessment, can be an important factor in reducing this risk factor.
- *Wandering or elopement.* Patients who are disoriented or suffering from cognitive disorders can be prone to wandering or elopement. Both of these events can pose a significant risk to older adult patients, particularly if the patient leaves the facility or if the wandering results in a fall. Organizations should put processes in place to assess and monitor patients who appear to pose a high wandering or elopement risk.
- *Magnetic Resonance Imaging (MRI).* Older adult patients may rely on assistive devices, and MRIs can produce dangerous levels of internal heating of the patient. Also, for those patients who have had any kind of passive implants, such as stints or shunts, they may contain magnetic or ferromagnetic elements that could be impacted by the MRI's magnetic effects. Organizations should plan to accommodate these risks by having transport devices or medical gases that are safe for use in the magnet room. Additional risk for older adult patients in MRI suites are for those patients with diminished renal function, which may predispose MRI patients to an increased risk of negative outcomes from MRI contrast agents containing gadolinium. As a result, older adult patients with compromised renal function should weigh the risks with their physicians. Organizations need to plan for this by assessing the patient before undergoing an MRI.[6]

Medical Equipment and Environmental Safety

The particular use or handling of certain medical equipment can have an impact on an older adult patient's safety. Also, how an environment is designed can have an impact on older adult patient safety. As has been discussed earlier in this chapter, older adult patients are at particular risk for such outcomes as falls, wandering, suicide, elopement, medication errors, and infections. All of these can be related to the environment or equipment.

The following represents some points of discussion in relation to medical equipment and environmental safety for organizations to consider.

Bed and toilet height. For older adult patients, the risk of falls is significant. Research indicates that seat height that is too high (more than 120% of lower leg length) or too low (less than 80% of lower leg length) can have an impact on safety and result in falls.[7] As an extrinsic risk factor, bed height needs to be in the lowest height possible to help prevent falls. Organizations should consider using adjustable beds left at the lowest setting for patients identified at high risk for falls to help reduce the chance and severity of falls.[8]

In the event that an organization is purchasing new beds, buying ones with a low-height setting may be beneficial for those patients at high risk. It has been customary for long term care settings to employ such measures for falls-risk patients. Another bed-related measure that may help reduce falls in the acute care setting is to lower bed height after any bedside procedures are done, in case the patient wishes to get out of bed but might be reluctant to adjust the bed him- or herself due to concern over staff inconvenience.[8]

Bedside safety rails. Bedside safety rails have often been used by health care organizations as a means to prevent patients from falling from their beds, and in some cases they are used as a restraint. Unfortunately, studies have found that the use of side rails has caused its own kind of adverse event, with their use being the cause of injury, and at times death, due to side-rail entrapment. Coupled with this is the finding that there is no evidence that the use of side rails actually plays a role in preventing falls.[9] In fact, one finding has indicated that rather than seeing the side rail as a protective or safety measure, some patients—especially those who may be suffering from poor cognitive ability—may simply view it as a barrier to go around. This makes the fall that a patient may suffer even worse, because climbing over the side rail can add up to 2 feet to the fall.[9] When deciding to reduce side rail use, organizations should not simply stop using them but need to come up with viable alternatives to their use. This can include improved assessment and monitoring techniques for those patients deemed at risk for falls or working with skilled staff, such as advance practice nurses, to devise alternative approaches to dealing with clinical problems that may have typically warranted the use of a side rail.

Bedside alarms. Some beds come equipped with bed alarms, which alert those nearby that the patient is moving out of the bed. These can be problematic, because in some cases alarms are not turned on or heard by staff.[10] Organizations should work on clear processes that encourage a consistent and manageable means to check on patients and ensure that their needs are met. In the case of alarms being unheard, it may be a better idea to move high-risk patients closer to the nurses' station so they can better hear the bed alarm and more frequently check on the patients.

Older adult patient safety-friendly equipment or features. Long term care settings have long known that it is not enough to simply ensure that bed heights are appropriate or that a falls-risk assessment is done to prevent falls among its residents. They also must ensure that the environment itself is suitable for their residents. Handrails along hallways, available walkers or canes, and placement of residents at risk for falls or wandering closer to the nurses' station for more frequent assessments can all be designed into the facility to help ensure that patients stay safe. Although a hospital is not going to exclusively admit older adult patients, the majority of its patients are going to be older adults. Organizations should work with their EC staff, nursing staff, and older adult specialists to ensure that any additional falls-reduction aids are in place to help patients successfully move without the increased chance of a fall.

Visual impairments. A common concern for older adult patients is visual decline. This can cause confusion, at the least, and adverse events, at the worst. To help older adult patients who might find a conventional organization's setting difficult to navigate due to diminishing eyesight, consider the following suggestions for implementation in your organization:[11]

- **Adequate signage size.** Signage should be large and have good contrast and wider spacing between characters.
- **Color contrast.** Consider using color contrasts that are easier for older adult patients to determine, such as yellows, oranges, and reds.
- **Depth perception.** Due to cataracts and other problems with depth perception, organizations should avoid floral or bold patterned carpeting on stairs.
- **Even lighting.** Even lighting can help reduce accents.
- **Glare should be reduced** to prevent visual problems.

Reduction of environmental triggers that might promote wandering. An identified best practice for reducing the incidence of wandering among older adult patients with dementia is reducing environmental triggers for wandering. M. Rowe, author of "Wandering in Hospitalized Older Adults," suggests the following interventions:[12]

- Avoid rooms near areas of high traffic or noise.
- Keep stars, elevators, and other exit cues out of the patient's view.
- Keep suitcases, shoes, and street clothes out of the patient's view.
- Position bed for best visibility and access to the bathroom; use orienting symbols to identify the bathroom (reds are most visible to the aging lens).

Special unit design. In the case of patients with dementia or other cognitive impairments, units should be designed with the following considerations in mind:[11]

- Avoid dead-end corridors. These have been found to cause agitation and frustration for dementia patients. Continuous walking tracks can be beneficial for wanderers.
- Consider using specific artwork as a visual cue for finding the way on the unit.
- Consider installing glare and flicker-free lighting.

Setting-Specific Physical Environment Concerns

Along with the complexity of issues that older adult patients may face, each health care setting faces its own unique challenges in relation to keeping an older adult patient safe. A home care agency caring for an older adult patient, for example, has to ensure that the patient's own home is safe for the patient who may face new and unexpected dangers, whereas a long term care facility can design its entire environment around care for the residents, most of whom are older adults. The following sections address some of the setting-specific issues that different health care settings may need to keep in mind in relation to older adult patient safety and the environment.

Hospitals

Older adult patients may spend less time in a hospital than in a long term care setting or in home care, but when under the care of a hospital they are generally much sicker and require far more medical care than in other settings. Also, due to the complexity of caring for an older adult patient, there is the increased risk of adverse events coming from what has been identified as the "hazards of hospitalization," of which some are clearly related to and can be impacted by, reduced by, or made worse by the environment:[13]

- Falls
- Restraint use
- Infection
- Delirium

Wandering and elopement are included as additional hazards in the hospital environment.

Some important issues to consider for older adult patients in a hospital setting include the following:

Be adaptive to older adult patients. A hospital may see many older adult patients, but that is not the only kind of patient it sees. As a result, it may not be financially feasible or realistic to make all units or departments specifically suited to an older adult patient. But adaptive measures can be introduced. Adjustable beds with low-height settings, additional hand rails, removal of room clutter, and bed alarms to signal movement by a patient who is at high risk for falls can all be introduced as environmental safeguards.

Home Care

Home care organizations face a special challenge of not only educating their older adult patients on patient safety issues but also helping assess the safety of the home environment. Particular areas of concern in home care include the following:

- *Falls:* Adequate lighting, clear pathways, safe floors (no scatter rugs)
- *Fire-related injuries:* Home fire extinguishers, more than one exit for safely departing from home, emergency plan to vacate the home, smoking, wood stove for heat

Due to the ongoing interaction that is in the nature of home care organizations, a visiting nurse or therapist has an opportunity to not only assess the safety of the home environment but also provide ongoing education for the older adult patient. If a patient has been discharged from the hospital into home care and was previously independent and in good health before the hospital visit, it may be a jarring experience for him or her to have to "make" his or her home safe. It may also be challenging for the patient's family to have to adapt to the changes in the home environment or to make an effort to ensure that the older adult patient manages risk. Patient and family education is a key intervention to help patients and families adapt their home to a safer environment.

Table 2-1 on page 24 includes a sample checklist that organizations can use to assess home safety.

Long Term Care

The long term care setting provides a significant number of challenges for ensuring older adult patient safety due to the population that it serves, though the specialized focus of those settings means that these organizations are often well positioned to prepare for risks. Long term care organizations face the following risks related to the environment:

- Falls
- Wandering or elopement
- Infection

In the case study on pages 25–27, one long term care organization, Perham Memorial Hospital and Home, located in Perham, Minnesota, shares its experiences of striking the balance between ensuring quality of life for its residents with excellent quality of care and safety when it had a recent opportunity to renovate and redesign its facility.

Emergency Management

Emergency management planning is a core component of any health care organization—organizations must plan and drill for the kinds of emergencies that can take place in their organization, be it responding to a natural disaster, such as a hurricane, or preparing for an influx of patients due to an epidemic. All populations that the health care organization serves

Table 2-1. Home Safety Checklist

Floor areas:

❑ Is the clutter clear or reduced?
❑ If there are throw rugs, have they been removed or moved?
❑ Are carpet edges secured?
❑ Have low-standing furniture and objects on the floor been removed?
❑ Have the cords and wires on the floor been removed?
❑ Have you checked lighting for adequate illumination at night?

Kitchen area:

❑ Are kitchen items easily within reach and manageable?
❑ Is there a step stool? If so, is it unsteady?
❑ Have chairs that are too low to sit on and/or stand up from easily been removed?

Bathrooms:

❑ Are grab bars installed in the bathtub or shower and by the toilet?
❑ Are rubber mats in the bathtub or shower?
❑ Is there a way to move up the floor mats when the bathtub or shower are not in use?
❑ Is a raised toilet seat installed?

Bedrooms:

❑ Is a light near the bed that can be easily reached?
❑ Has adequate lighting been installed in the bedroom?
❑ Is the bedroom easily accessible?

Outdoors:

❑ Is the shrubbery trimmed along the pathway to the home?
❑ Has adequate lighting been installed by doorways and long walkways leading to doors?
❑ As feasible, are sidewalks or pathways safe to walk and cracks reduced?
❑ Are handrails on outdoor stairs and steps?

Stairs and steps:

❑ Are stairs free of clutter?
❑ Have any loose or uneven steps been repaired?
❑ Are handrails on both sides of the stairs?
❑ Are handrails on staircases installed?

Other safety tips:

❑ Are emergency numbers in large print near each phone?
❑ If there is a cell phone, have emergency numbers been programmed in?
❑ Is a fire alarm installed in the home?
❑ Has a phone been placed near the floor in the event of a fall?
❑ Has the patient considered wearing a fall alert device for help in the event of a fall?

CASE STUDY

Situated 65 miles east of Fargo, North Dakota, Perham Memorial Hospital and Home is a 96-bed skilled long term care organization located in Perham, Minnesota. Perham serves a rural community and has limited funds for major renovations or building work. But in 2000, money was allocated to begin a renovation of its nursing home.

Marilyn Oelfke, R.N., senior director of long term care services and director of nursing of Perham Memorial Hospital and Home, describes how the nursing home began its improvement process and credits her feeling that the improvement project got off to the right start to the hospital and home's leadership. "Our [chief executive officer], Chuck Hofius, suggested that before we actually went ahead and renovated the home to resemble what we had beforehand, we take the time to see if anything else would be more helpful," Oelfke explains.

Designing Change

In 2000, the nursing home was a 102-bed facility consisting of 32-bed units. "We had good satisfaction rates and were well regarded in the community," notes Oelfke. "We provided excellent quality of care." But when Perham asked its staff if they were ready to move into the existing nursing home, no one was ready to do so. If the nursing home wasn't ready for staff, changes needed to be made for the next generation of elders. This became a challenge for Perham. "We decided to listen to our own feedback and create a nursing home that anyone would be happy with," Oelfke continues.

After careful consideration of innovative models in long term care that provide a high quality of life in nursing homes while ensuring quality and safety of care, Perham decided to adopt the household model and use that as the guiding principle for its renovation work. The household model promotes residents living in smaller "households" with other residents and a dedicated staff. The model also promotes more resident-directed care with residents having more control over how they live in the setting.

Perham wanted to ensure quality of care while balancing it with quality of life. "We wanted to provide the residents with control over how they lived in the home," explains Oelfke. So the focus of the redesign was on how to provide that goal for its residents. Perham opted to build new, replacing 64 beds in the old building with four households of 16 residents each. Two of the existing units were then remodeled into 16-bed households, with the final unit remodeled into the "town center." The town center includes a chapel, shop, café, theater, and beauty/barber shop. Each household has its own kitchen, living room, laundry, and dining room, and residents are able to determine when they want to get up or go to bed, what they want to eat, and how they spend their time.

The Redesign: Facility Remodel and Staff Training

Working with experts in the household model, Perham wasted no time in orienting and training staff on the new approach, which included one fairly important and potentially challenging change for staff: All staff would be cross-trained in each other's jobs. The household approach had permanent staff attached to each household, so all staff had to know how to do the work of caring for residents, including such areas as nutrition, housekeeping, nurse assistance, and activities. Oelfke notes that the goal of all household staff being cross-trained is simple: "Everyone in the household should be able to answer lights and respond to the residents' needs."

"Orientation began as the physical renovation was underway." Oelfke says. "We knew that making this new

At-a-Glance

About the long term care organization: Perham Memorial Hospital and Home, located in Perham, Minnesota, serves a rural community with skilled nursing for 96 beds in its long term care facility, attached to its hospital.

About the improvement: When Perham Memorial Hospital and Home began planning to renovate its long term care facility, leadership realized that it faced a unique opportunity to completely reconsider how it would design and rebuild its facility with its residents in mind.

approach work meant a culture change for staff, and that takes time." Perham also focused on training staff in communication skills, problem solving, and working on self-directed teams. Oelfke sees all this training as an important and necessary component of establishing the culture of change that would allow the home to provide excellent care while ensuring quality of life. "Our true focus is on striking a balance between quality of care and quality of life," notes Oelfke. "Our goal is to create a home for our residents where they have choice and control over how they will live and what they will do." Safety was also an important factor in how the home was redesigned but was kept in balance with the goal of retaining quality of life. Even before the physical remodel was done, the home began following its new household model in 2004.

Oelfke describes some aspects of the physical redesign: "We designed shorter halls, added carpet, installed a wireless call system, put in measures to reduce noise in the environment, designed measures to reduce traffic through the households, and added nonskid flooring in bathrooms." By late 2006, the new building (the town center) was complete, and the households were physically in place. As the home had spent the previous 2 years adapting to the new model, it was easier for residents and staff to seamlessly adapt to their new surroundings.

A New Model: A New Home

For Oelfke, the most dramatic change she has observed since the redesign of Perham is in the way that residents are in the home. "It used to be that one might see a nursing home as a place to come and die," Oelfke says. "In the old model, we were so concerned about doing everything possible for the residents that in some ways we inadvertently took their lives away. Now, in the new model, the residents are truly living."

"We engage residents in all aspects of their care," explains Oelfke. "They tell us what they want their routine to be, and we adapt to them." As a result, Oelfke has seen a dramatic reduction in residents resisting care, resulting in less injury to staff and residents alike. "We've also noticed a reduction in reliance on psychotropic medications," she continues.

Residents are involved not only in decision making relating to their own care but in life at the home. "Residents are invited to attend household council meetings and share concerns directly with staff," Oelfke says. "Residents are also involved in selecting staff. By being able to choose and invite staff into their home, the residents feel more secure with new staff, as they are not strangers to them."

Residents are also encouraged to participate in safety efforts. "We currently have a falls team meeting in the home," says Oelfke. "We did circle meetings in each household with our residents to find out their concerns related to falls; we asked them to share their own thoughts on why they fall and what we all can do differently to help prevent falls." The feedback has been helpful and is being integrated into ongoing improvement efforts to prevent falls.

Learning from Experience

Oelfke offers the following advice to other long term care organizations hoping to adopt a new approach to providing care to their residents:

- *Make sure that everyone is onboard for the change.* Because this kind of change requires support from all levels of the organization, engage staff in the process early and consistently.
- *Adopt a learning approach.* Visit other facilities that have undertaken a similar approach and do your research.
- *Educate, educate, educate.* Create an atmosphere of learning; embrace the concept of a learning "blame-free" work environment where the focus is on the system and not the person.
- *Involve residents and families early and often.* Let residents and families know what is happening and gain their support and feedback at every step along the way.
- *Get comfortable talking.* Get used to encouraging staff and residents to sit together to share successes and failures. This is an important aspect of resident-centered care and ensuring residents are engaged in their own safety.
- *Be patient with the process.* Go slowly. Change of this kind is evolutionary, not revolutionary.
- *Rely on strong leadership.* Consider everyone as leaders. Formal leaders need to "model the way," but encourage

and empower staff members to own the process and add their perspective and experience to it.

- *Keep the focus on the residents.* Residents and resident-centered care should be the focus of all improvement efforts.
- *Do not be afraid of cross-training.* Although cross-training can be challenging for some staff to get used to, don't be afraid to try it and help staff adapt to the new approach. "[This] is one of the primary steps that really changes the culture of how we work," says Oelfke.

Lessons Learned

Oelfke shares the following lessons that Perham learned along the way as they redesigned their home:

- Do not take on too much, too quickly; let staff and residents set the pace.
- For new buildings, allow staff who will be working in the new areas adequate time to set up the area before moving into it.
- Keep in mind that residents can and do contribute in meaningful ways to ensure quality of care, quality of life, and safety.
- It is important to learn that families play a significant role in the households.
- By focusing on improving residents' quality of life, Oelfke notes that Perham has seen the quality of care improve well beyond what they could have imagined. "We're seeing a reduction in the use of psychotropic medications, better pain control, fewer pressure ulcers, fewer medication errors, physically stronger residents, a reduced risk of choking, weight gain among residents, a reduction in the reliance on supplements, and less anxiety and depression among residents." Perhaps most striking and encouraging to staff at Perham, Oelfke notes that they are seeing a renewed spirit and engagement in life among residents.

There can be added costs, a need for more education and training, and possibly more building work required when renovating a nursing home to a new model of care, but for Perham, the costs have been well worth it. "One result from these changes that we never expected to see was that people really 'choose' to stay here now," states Oelfke. "With the old nursing home model, residents were often fearful of what might happen to them and most likely accepted it with a sense of resignation, but now residents love being here, and we even have a large waiting list for the home."

must be taken into consideration when planning for an emergency. Some populations are particularly vulnerable, and in some settings, planning for their needs in an emergency is particularly complicated. In the case of older adult patients, special concerns should be considered when planning for emergencies.

Older Adult Concerns During an Emergency

Any time an emergency hits a community, health care organizations have to respond effectively in stressful and chaotic situations. They often have to tend to patients who are vulnerable and compromised. Simply ordering patients to "leave the building" is not enough.

In the case of older adult patients, it can be helpful to be mindful of their vulnerabilities when planning for an emergency. Consider what happened during Hurricane Katrina in 2005, a recent disaster that teaches some important lessons about what can happen for older adult patients during an emergency.

In 2006, the Department of Health and Human Services reported on the emergency preparedness and response of a select number of nursing homes in the Gulf states after Hurricane Katrina. This devastating natural disaster tested the ability of health care organizations throughout the region to respond and cope, and in the case of long term care organizations, it raised some important issues regarding how to respond to the needs of older adult patients in a crisis.[14]

The report found that in those cases in which residents of a long term care facility were evacuated, there was a higher incidence of depression, skin tears, and dehydration than in those facilities where residents were not evacuated.[14] Even in the case of those facilities that did not evacuate, the long term care facilities reported problems with staffing, maintaining supplies, and facility services. However, the decision to evacuate or stay is not always in the hands of the organization, because it can often be imposed on an organization by community evacuation orders; therefore, organizations need to be prepared for either situation, because they can all pose a risk to the safety and well being of residents.[14] Additional problems related to transportation, complications with medications, inadequate staffing or facilities at the evacuation location, and insufficient food and water were experienced. The report also found that those organizations that did evacuate experienced problems with re-entry to the organization.

In a survey focused on long term care facilities in Texas during Hurricanes Katrina and Rita in August and September 2005, organizations reported that deaths did occur among residents during evacuations, along with financial losses due to staffing overtime and transportation needs. As with the report on the long term care facilities throughout the Gulf states, the Texas study noted that whether evacuated or not, organizations faced similar challenges. It also reported that organizations felt that they needed to improve their training for emergency preparedness and needed to be prepared for the unexpected developments that come about during natural disasters.[15] In the case of the events of 2005, while the region was just beginning to recover from the advent of Katrina, Hurricane Rita approached, leaving states like Texas bowed under the pressure of having just received 450,000 evacuees and now having to cope with a second hurricane, making it difficult for health care organizations to implement emergency plans that had not anticipated the fact that they would have just received a significant number of residents or patients.

If anything is to be learned from what happened in 2005, it would be that although emergency plans are crucial for organizations to have on hand, drafting those plans and doing the occasional drills may not be enough. One area of concern raised by the U.S. Department of Health and Human Services (HHS) in its 2006 report was the finding that many long term care administrators noted that, because of the many complexities that came from the disaster, they were forced to deviate from their actual emergency plan or had to cope with unanticipated elements.[14] These unanticipated elements resulted in some near misses for residents. In addition, issues related to evacuation routes came up as recurring challenges. So it may be worth considering spending more time training staff for the variety of challenges that could be faced in an emergency.

Planning for Different Types of Emergencies

There is no way to plan for every type of emergency that can impact a health care organization, though careful planning and consideration can help an organization plan for what may be the most common types of emergencies facing that organization. Plans should accommodate whether evacuation will take place, what type of public health disaster could hit them (for example, an outbreak of influenza), what type of natural disasters affect their geographical area (tornados, flooding, hurricanes), and what kinds of community planning should take place.

Consider the following tips when planning for different types of emergencies in relation to older adult patients:

Prepare for the most vulnerable patients. If you care for very vulnerable patients, planning for their needs in the event of evacuation or loss of power due to an emergency, for example, can help you plan for most situations. If you have older adult patients with special needs, such as oxygen or feeding tubes, you should have systems in place to care for them regardless of relocation or being sheltered in place.

Continue to assess for older adult-related risk. In a hectic environment where staff and patients are impacted by the emergency that is underway, it can be easy to neglect the fundamental assessments and monitoring that might otherwise be ongoing. Emergency plans should include provisions for staff to ensure that the changed surroundings do not pose an additional risk for older adult patients, such as in the case of falls or pressure ulcers.

Supplies. Supplies are an essential necessity for any health care organization. Depending on the setting (with long term care organizations needing more, for example), older adult patients will often need such supplies as prescription medications, special dietary supplies, and so on. If patients are sheltered within the organization, general supplies will also be required, such as water, canned food, generators, and so on. In the case of home care organizations, patients will need to be educated on what to have available at home in the event of an emergency.[15] The 2006 HHS report noted that some supplies were not as accessible to organizations during the hurricane. Organizations should take stock of their supplies and ensure that they have sufficient supplies available during an emergency. Smaller organizations may benefit from collaborating with other nearby organizations to pool resources.

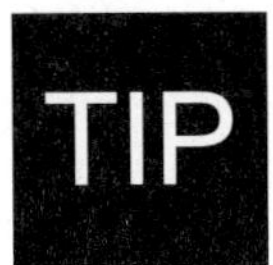

Community and interorganization collaboration. Health care organizations need to interface with the community to help plan for a possible influx of patients and how to educate the community on what to do in the event of an emergency, and to collaborate on essential services during an emergency. If residents of a long term care facility have to be evacuated due to an emergency in the facility, for example, emergency preparedness should plan for where the residents should be relocated, which may be within the community or in a nearby facility.

Conclusion

Older adult patients can face particular needs in relation to the environment of physical care, where the very environment they are in can make a significant difference in how safe they are. This can be particularly challenging in the case of residents of long term care facilities, where they may be receiving skilled nursing care, but they are also living in the facility—a balance must be struck between providing excellent quality of care and safety and quality of life. In the case of older adult patients who receive ambulatory or home care, educating the patient in ensuring his or her home environment is safe can have an impact on reducing adverse events, such as falls. The measures health care organizations put in place in their environment can play an important role in ensuring that patients not only receive high-quality care but also remain safe in their surroundings. The following chapter, Chapter 3, explores issues of medication safety for older adult patients.

References

1. Gold M.F.: Designs for extended living. *Provider*, pp. 18–26, Nov. 2004.
2. Redman R.W.: Practice environments: Cognitive aspects of adverse events. *Res Theory Nurs Prac* 21(1):10–12, 2007.
3. Rabig J., et al.: Radical re-design of nursing homes: Applying the green house concept in Tupelo, MS. *Gerontologist* 46:534–539, 2006.
4. Kane R.A., et al.: Resident outcomes in small-house nursing homes: A longitudinal evaluation of the initial green house Program. *J Am Geriatr Soc* 55(6):832–839, Jun. 2007.
5. The Green House® Concept. http://www.ncbcapitalimpact.org/default.aspx?id=148 (accessed Feb. 19, 2009).
6. Evaluating MRI safety for specific populations. *Jt Comm J Qual Patient Saf* 7:5–11, June 2007.
7. Capezuti E., et al.: Bed and toilet height as potential environmental risk factors. *Clin Nurs Res* 17:50–66, Feb. 2008.
8. Tzeng H.M., Yin C.Y.: Height of hospital beds and inpatient falls: A threat to patient safety. *J Nurs Admin* 37:537–538, Dec. 2007.
9. Capezuti E., et al.: Consequences of an intervention to reduce restrictive side rail use in nursing homes. *J Am Geriatr Soc* 55:334–341, Mar. 2007.
10. Tzeng H.M., Yin C.Y.: Nurses' solutions to prevent inpatient falls in hospital patient rooms. http://findarticles.com/p/articles/mi_m0FSW/is_3_26/ai_n27871615/pg_8 (accessed Feb. 19, 2009).
11. Wang C.H., Kuo N.W.: Zeitgeists and development trends in long-term care facility design. *J Nurs Res* 14(2):123–128, 2006.
12. Rowe M.: Wandering in hospitalized older adults. *Am J Nurs* 18:62–70, Oct. 2008.
13. Fernandez H.M., et al.: House staff member awareness of older inpatients' risk for hazards of hospitalization. *Arch Intern Med* 168:390–396, Feb. 25, 2008.
14. Department of Health and Services: Office of Inspector General. *Nursing Home Emergency Preparedness and Response During Recent Hurricanes.* http://www.oig.hhs.gov/oei/reports/oei-06-06-00020.pdf (accessed Feb. 19, 2009).
15. Castro C., et al.: Surviving the storms: Emergency preparedness in texas nursing facilities and assisted living facilities. *J Geriatr Nurs* 34(8):9–16, 2008.

Chapter 3

Medication Safety for Older Adults

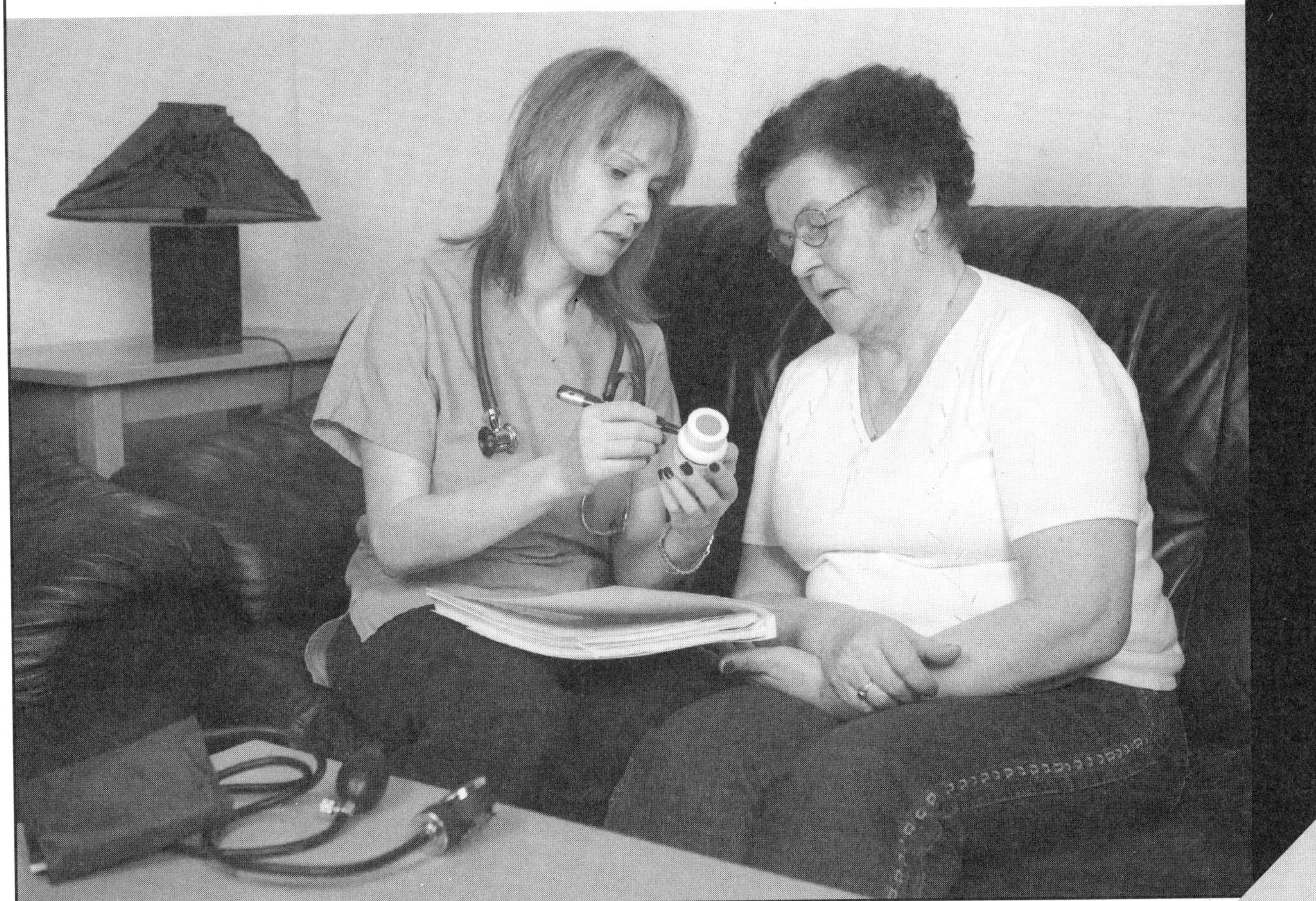

For many older adult patients, using medications on a daily basis is a way of life. Due to the complexity of conditions that older adult patients face, they will often be asked to adhere to a complicated medication regimen. Although older adult patients are the largest users of prescription medication, their advancing age will often make them more vulnerable to adverse reactions to the medications they are taking. A full 30% of older adult patient hospital admissions are drug related, with 11% attributed to medication nonadherence and 10% to 17% related to adverse drug reactions (ADRs).[1] The Joint Commission reports that medication errors represent 8.7% of sentinel events reported, with only suicide and post-operative or operative complications being higher.[2]

The following represent the most frequent kinds of medication-related errors:[3]

- Taking an unauthorized drug
- Taking the wrong dose
- Missing a dose/not completing a regimen
- Taking a dose at the wrong time
- Taking an extra dose
- Continuing a drug after it is discontinued
- Inappropriate use of a medication
- Giving a drug to the wrong patient
- Giving a drug via the wrong route
- Incorrectly diluting a drug
- Inappropriately administrating a drug

Often reported causes of medication errors include the following:[3]

- Polypharmacy
- Knowledge deficits (patient and/or caregiver)
- Transcription errors/errors in communication
- Confusion over hospital discharge instruction (patient and/or clinician)
- Confusion over brand name versus generic name
- Medications that look alike or sound alike
- Incorrect use of medication boxes
- Skipped doses due to cost, fear of side effects, lack of transportation to pharmacy
- Cognitive and visual problems

Effective medication management is a crucial patient safety strategy for any health care organization, and in the case of older adult patients, particular risks require focused attention: polypharmacy, nonadherence to medication, and ADRs. All these events can lead to problems for older adult patients that can result in unintended admissions to hospitals or admission to long term care facilities. Organizations should consider how they will assess an older adult patient's use of medications, provide ongoing assessment and education, and ensure that they understand the connections between certain medication use and increased safety risks, such as falls. Additional risk factors facing older adult patients include living alone, impaired vision, impaired cognitive function, being age 75 and over, having three or more medications and/or scheduled doses in 1 day, and more than one prescribing provider.[1] This chapter discusses some of the biggest medication-related challenges older adult patients face and addresses some possible solutions for organizations to consider.

In the Notes from the Field on page 33, Elaine Buccellato discusses safe medication practices for older adult patients.

Medication Risks and Safety for Older Adults

We live in a time of contrasts. The ever-growing number of effective therapeutic treatments has allowed those of advancing age to enjoy healthier, longer lives. But the irony is that those same therapeutic treatments can cause problems for patients as well.

Polypharmacy

Polypharmacy, or the use of multiple medications by a patient, is a common occurrence among older adult patients. This often results from older adult patients seeing a variety of physicians for a number of ailments, resulting in that older adult patient often being on a disproportionate number of prescriptions. Fully 40% of people over the age of 65 use 5 or more different medications, and 12% use more than 10.[4] Although polypharmacy will not pose a high risk for all patients nor will all medications have an unsafe drug-drug interaction, especially if their medication use is being carefully monitored and reviewed and found to be clinically appropriate, but it has been found to be one of the risk factors for older adult patients.[5]

When an older adult patient takes an increasing number of medications, it can increase the risk of drug interaction and ADEs. Health care providers need to work carefully to

Notes from the Field: Safe Medication Practices for Older Adults

Joint Commission surveyor Elaine Buccellato, R.N., B.S.N., M.S., stresses the importance of safe medication practices in relation to older adult patients. Most older adult patients are on multiple medications, and when hospitalized this list usually increases over time. The use of multiple pharmacies increases the possibility of adverse drug events (ADEs). Continuity of care is especially important when medication information is transferred from "one caregiver to another" or from "one facility to another." Therefore, another medication-related area of safety concern for health care organizations is to ensure that the older adult patient's medications are reconciled across the continuum accurately. "Organizations need to implement safe practices to reconcile medications when older adult patients are admitted or discharged from their organizations. Staff needs to work carefully with older adult patients to help them identify all their medications," Buccellato says. She states, "Geriatric patients, on admission and discharge, need particular guidance on identifying home medications and can often forget to mention certain medications, such as over-the-counter eye drops, vitamins, and pain medications."

"Communication between staff and patients in relation to their medication use is crucial," she notes. Because many geriatric patients face complex medication regimens, Buccellato states that "it is very important that things are communicated clearly to the geriatric patient. Patients themselves can be important assets in patient safety. I was visiting a health care organization where I observed the geriatric patient telling the nurse, 'I don't get a green pill,' and the patient was right. This drives home the importance of patients being involved in their care and medication education." Buccellato adds, "In that situation, if the resident had never been educated or empowered to point out mistakes, then there could have been a potential adverse outcome. A geriatric patient has an important role to play in his or her own safety."

ensure that the number and combination of drugs are beneficial and safe for the patient. This can be more easily managed if the patient is only seeing one care provider or his or her care is managed in a multidisciplinary, collaborative manner. When a patient is receiving care from multiple providers or has been transitioning between multiple care settings, breakdowns in communication can occur, and knowledge about medications taken may be lost or poorly communicated. It can often be assumed that the patient him- or herself will be responsible for tracking his or her own medications, but that may be unrealistic. Also, because some older adult patients may not consider over-the-counter medications, supplements, or herbal remedies to be medication, they may underreport what they are taking.

The times when polypharmacy can pose a heightened risk to a patient include if the patient is over age 75, is seeing multiple providers, or is on a complicated polypharmacy regimen. If a patient, for example, is taking multiple medications at different times of the day, it can be confusing to keep track of which medication is taken when and could result in nonadherence or an adverse event.

Consider the following tips for minimizing the risks of adverse events resulting from polypharmacy:

Use the "brown bag" technique. Ambulatory care organizations can take advantage of ongoing visits by having older adult patients bring in all their medications—including over-the-counter and herbal supplements—during a doctor's visit for assessment. Other settings can also benefit from this.

Encourage patients to understand their own medications. Patients have a key role to play in their own safety. Use patient education and mentoring techniques to teach patients what their medications do, what they are named, what to do if they miss a dose, why they are taking them, and what their side effects can be. They should also know how to communicate with their providers if there are any adverse events.

Sidebar 3-1. Tips to Minimize Patient Risk of Adverse Reactions When Taking Multiple Drugs (Polypharmacy)

Know your medications:

- What are their names?
- Why are you taking them?
- How should your drugs be taken?
- What are their most common and most serious side effects?
- What should you do if problems arise?
- What should you do if you miss a dose?
- If you have been in the hospital, do you know what you should be taking when you are discharged? (Many changes may have been made to your medications during your hospital stay. When discharged, it is important for you to know what you should be taking.)

Communicate with your doctor and pharmacist:

- Tell your doctor and pharmacist about all the drugs you are taking, including over-the-counter drugs, dietary supplements, and herbal remedies.
- Do not expect a "pill for every ill." Some health concerns will go away without treatment or be better managed by therapies other than drugs. Discuss with your doctor how best to deal with your health concerns and consider all treatment options.
- Inform your doctor about any allergies or reactions you have had to drugs in the past.
- Tell your doctor about any problems that develop after starting a new drug.
- Do not stop taking a prescribed drug without talking it over with your doctor. Before starting an over-the-counter agent, supplement, or herbal remedy, check with your doctor or pharmacist to ensure that it will be safe to take.

Be organized:

- Keep an up-to-date written list of all the drugs, dietary supplements, and herbal remedies you are taking.
- When you see your doctor, be prepared. Before the visit, think about what you want to talk about and write it down if necessary.
- Periodically review your list of drugs and over-the-counter products with your doctor. Ask whether it is necessary for you to continue taking everything on the list.
- Take your medications as directed.
- Do not share your drugs.
- Do not save prescribed drugs for future use "just in case" unless you are asked to do so by your doctor. Do not keep old medications (check the expiration date on the pill bottle).
- Store your drugs in a secure, dry place out of sunlight. Find out if your medications should be refrigerated.
- Use devices (for example, a blister pack or 7-day pill organizer) to help you take your drugs as directed.
- It is generally better to have one physician prescribing and one pharmacy dispensing your medications. This makes it easier for your doctor and pharmacist to watch for potential adverse reactions between drugs.

Source: *Hogan D.B., Kwan M.: Tips for avoiding problems with polypharmacy.* Can Med Assoc J, *Oct. 10, 2006. http://www.cmaj.ca/content/vol175/issue8/ (accessed Mar. 23, 2009).*

Make sure the regimen is necessary and as simple as possible. Research has found that increased complexity in a polypharmacy regimen can make it more difficult for patients to follow the regimen or can increase the chance of a medication error. If medication is found to not be therapeutic or a better alternative is available, consider a new approach. Duplicate medications should be avoided, if possible. Organizations should put measures in place to ensure they review a patient's medication and that the regimen is as straightforward as possible for a patient to follow.

Work with advanced practitioners. It could be a huge benefit for an organization if it works with advanced practitioners, such as elder care pharmacists or gerontological nurse practitioners, to review medication use and, if necessary, work to help change the therapies to a safer, more manageable combination.

Table 3-1. Poor Adherence Checklist

Predictor of Poor Adherence	Organization-Identified Risk Factors in Population Served
Presence of psychological problems (for example, depression)	
Presence of cognitive impairment	
Treatment of asymptomatic disease	
Inadequate follow-up or discharge planning	
Side effect of medication	
Patient's lack of belief in benefits of treatment	
Patient's lack of insight into the illness	
Non-Caucasian	
Poor provider-patient relationship	
Presence of barriers to care or medications	
Missed appointments	
Complexity of treatment	
Cost of medication, copayment, or both	

Sidebar 3-1, page 34, contains tips for how patients can be engaged in their own polypharmacy safety.

Medication Nonadherence

Medication nonadherence, when a patient does not follow the instructions given for taking a prescribed medication, poses a risk for older adult patients, either by worsening their condition (due to not taking the medication) or by potentially triggering an adverse drug interaction (due to taking the medication incorrectly). Medication nonadherence has been linked to having multiple providers, with those patients with more than three chronic conditions being less adherent to taking their medicine.[6] Medication nonadherence can also be linked directly to patient behaviors and a patient's perception of his or her medications. On the one hand, a patient may not remember when to take a dose, may mix up medicines, or may have misunderstood the provided instructions; and on the other hand, a patient may not feel certain of the medicines' effectiveness or worth. For example, a patient might not believe that he or she could take the medicine as described (impractical dosing, concern over side effects), might not see the necessity of the medicine, might be unsure as to the medicine's effectiveness, or might be concerned that the medicine's possible adverse effects could outweigh the benefit.[7]

The following includes a list of some of the major predictors of poor adherence to medication:[8]

- Presence of psychological problems (for example, depression)
- Presence of cognitive impairment
- Treatment of asymptomatic disease
- Inadequate follow-up or discharge planning
- Side effect of medication
- Patient's lack of belief in benefits of treatment
- Patient's lack of insight into the illness
- Non-Caucasian
- Poor provider-patient relationship
- Presence of barriers to care or medications
- Missed appointments
- Complexity of treatment
- Cost of medication, copayment, or both

Sidebar 3-2. A Nine-Step Office-Based Approach to Improving Medication Adherence

To help his older patients deal with the compound issues of polypharmacy and their well-documented nonadherence, Fredrick T. Sherman, M.D., M.Sc., professor of geriatrics and medicine, the Brookdale Department of Geriatrics and Adult Development, Mount Sinai School of Medicine, and medical director for Senior Health Partners, New York, has an active dialogue during the office visit, addressing as many of these nine points as time will allow:

1. Have older adults to bring all their medications with them to each visit (the "brown-bag" test), or at least a medication list.

   Primary care physicians, however, should be cautious about the accuracy of the brown-bag test. A study of community-residing patients (average age 79) compared the medications these seniors actually brought to their clinic visit (they were told on multiple occasions to bring "all their medications") with those that were found when a physician performed an in-home medication inspection, searching room to room for all medications. The in-home assessment revealed that half of all patients had omitted at least one regular medicine and that one-fifth had omitted a prescribed medicine.

2. Ask older adults how they take each of their medications, and then to open a vial, take out the actual number of pills, and close the vial. This helps assess both their understanding of what's written on the medication vials and their ability to self-administer their medicines in either the non–child-resistant or child-resistant vials.

3. If patients are using hard-to-open, child-resistant vials and have difficulty opening them, ask them whether they actually need these vials (that is, if they live in a three-generation household with grandchildren) or whether they would prefer easy-to-open non–child-resistant vials. If the latter is the case, tell them to ask their pharmacist. Alternatively, write on their prescription "Dispense in non–child-resistant containers."

4. Ask patients if they are having problems paying for their medicines. Are they trying to save money by not filling prescriptions, skipping doses, or taking smaller doses? If so, make sure to prescribe generics or less-expensive brands.

5. If adding or deleting a medication, make sure that patients understand the change.

6. If patients are taking four or more chronic medications, recommend that they use a time-specific dosing pack, such as a plastic or a disposable punch card blister pack or an egg box that has been filled with the patient's weekly medicines. In a recent randomized controlled trial of 200 community-based patients age 65 and older taking nine chronic medications, the combination of standardized medication education, regular follow-up by a pharmacist, and medications dispensed in time-specific packs (blister packs) increased medication adherence from 61% to 97%. Remarkably, the proportion of seniors who achieved greater than 80% adherence for all their medications increased by 16-fold, from 5% to 99%.

7. Use a once-daily regimen with long-acting medications. If compliance is a problem, prescribe a combination tablet to minimize the number of doses and drugs that have to be remembered.

8. Because the number of medications older adults take has probably doubled in the past decade, keep the medication list as simple as possible, stopping all medications that are no longer indicated and tapering all medications whose therapeutic efficacy is questionable.

9. Start low and go slow with a newly added medicine, being prepared to go high with the dosage and pushing to therapeutic efficacy while avoiding toxicity.

Although these nine steps may seem like a lot to do during each office visit, using a check-off list will enhance efficiency. Alternatively, an office nurse can review many of these steps with the elderly patient and the family, if needed, at the conclusion of the office visit.

Source: *Sherman F.T.: Medicational nonadherence: A national epidemic among America's seniors.* Geriatrics *62:5–6, Apr. 2007.*

To determine if your patients are at risk for poor adherence, consider completing the checklist in Table 3-1—based on the aforementioned list—as a starting point to plan improvements.

One study of chronically ill people starting a new medication found that almost one-third did not take their medications as prescribed, and of that one-third, 50% were deliberately nonadherent.[9] This kind of intentional nonadherence is related to older adult patients' perception of their illness and concern over being vulnerable to complications related to the medication. In fact, the bulk of research indicates that patients skip doses due to side effects.[9] Other reasons for nonadherence can be financial, where a patient simply cannot afford the prescribed medication. If a patient feels free to express such a concern to his or her provider, it may be possible to suggest less-expensive generic alternatives. Research also indicates that those patients who have open and clear lines of communication with their provider, along with education and mentoring for improved self-management, tend to have higher adherence rates.

In trying to reduce the incidence of nonadherence among older adult patients, organizations should work on improving and honing their communication with patients. Consider the tips in Sidebar 3-2 on page 36 on effectively communicating with patients to improve their medication adherence.

Consider using the strategies in Sidebar 3-3, right, to improve medication adherence among older adult patients.

Sidebar 3-3. Possible Strategies to Improve Medication Adherence in Older Adult Patients

Behavioral

- Use of a pillbox or calendar pack
- Reminder chart/medication list
- Reminders (mail, telephone, e-mail)
- E-mail education and training
- Self-medication training by health care provider
- Skill building (supervised, group)
- Tailoring (routinization)
- Adherence monitoring/feedback (obtrusive pill count, medication monitor)
- Alarm/beeper use
- Cell phone or PDA reminder
- Calendar/diary
- Contracting (verbal or written agreement)
- Large-print labels
- Packaging change
- Follow up (home visit, scheduled clinic visit, video/teleconferencing)

Education (by health care organization)

- Group education, in a warfarin clinic, for example (inpatient, family, group)
- Individualized (use of oral, audiovisual, visual, written, telephone, mail processes)

Staff training

- Education (on site, workshops, in-services)
- Mentoring
- Medication literature review

High-Alert Medications and Drug-Drug Interactions for Older Adult Patients

Considering the fact that older adult patients take more medications and are more prone to ADEs than their younger counterparts, organizations have to be hyperaware of the kinds of medications that can increase risk. Research points to a number of high-alert medications that require special attention. In the case of older adult patients, extra care should be taken to ensure that any additional drugs are taken into consideration when prescribing.

Medications can also factor into increased safety risk for older adult patients, particularly in relation to disorientation or falls. Older adult patients are particularly vulnerable to orthostatic hypotension because of age-related changes in baraoreceptor reflex sensibility. Certain antihypertensive medications, for example, can lower blood pressure but thereby increase the incidence of falls risk, such as the following:[10]

- Alpha-adrenegic blockers
- Angiotensin-converting enzyme inhibitors
- Anticholinergics
- Antidepressants
- Antiparkinsonian agents

Table 3-2. Common Drug Interactions

Primary Drug...	Interacting With...	Potential Effect...
Digoxin	St. John's wort	Plasma concentration of digoxin reduced
Griseofulvin	Warfarin	Anticoagulant effect reduced
Lithium	Many analgesics	Lithium excretion reduced
Nitrates	Sildenafil	Hypotensive effect increased
Simvastin	Itraconazole Ketoconazole	Increased risk of myopathy
Sulphonylureas	Antifungals	Increased risk of hypoglycemia
Warfarin	Many antibiotics	Anticoagulation may be increased

Source: *Institute for Safe Medication Practices. http://www.ismp.org (accessed Mar. 23, 2009).*

- Antipsychotics
- Beta-blockers
- Nitrates
- Opioids
- Phosphodiesterase type-5 inhibitors
- Skeletal muscle relaxants

Drug combinations can also cause unexpected reactions in older adult patients, and due to their higher rates of polypharmacy, they are at even higher risks of facing unexpected drug interactions. The following constitute some dangerous drug combinations that organizations should be aware of:

- If Phosphodiesterase type-5 inhibitors (used for erectile dysfunction) are used with nitrates or antihypertensives, this combination can increase hypotensive effects.
- If benzodiazepines (such as clonazepam) are used with azole antifungals (such as ketoconazole), benzodiazepine and enhanced sedation can result from the combination.
- If macrolide antibiotics (erythromycin) are combined with digoxin, the combination can cause increased serum digoxin levels, with altered mental status, visual disturbances, hypotension, and dizziness.[10]

Additional drug interactions that can increase safety risks for older adult patients are listed in Table 3-2.

Certain drugs or drug groups need special consideration in relation to older adult patient safety. They include the following:[9]

- *Anticoagulants.* These can cause excessive anticoagulation and can increase an older adult patient's risk for bleeding. Some medications interact with anticoagulants and raise bleeding risks by increasing the internationalized normalized ratio, and certain foods, if not eaten in consistent amounts, can also negatively impact the effectiveness of the anticoagulants. Patients need to be monitored closely and carefully educated on the risks.
- *Antipsychotics, anxiolytics, antidepressants, and sedatives.* All of these medicines can have the opposite impact on older adult patients. These drugs can all have a negative impact on falls risk.
- *Antihypertensive drugs.* These drugs can cause hypokalemia, hyperglycemia, and hyperuricemia, all dangerous conditions for older adult patients who could suffer from diabetes, arrhythmia, and gout.

- *Antimicrobials.* Due to decreased renal clearance in older adult patients, kidney-extracted antimicrobials have a longer half-life.
- *Cardiac glycosides.* These preparations, such as digoxin, are commonly prescribed to older adults for atrial fibrillation and heart failure. But due to age-related decreases in Glomerular filtration rates, an older adult patient is susceptible to risks of digoxin toxicity.
- *Certain over-the-counter medicines.* Aspirin can cause salicylate toxicity; antacids can interfere with other medications and cause hypercalcemia and renal stones or failure; laxatives can compromise a patient's nutritional status, if used chronically.

Based on this information, organizations should work toward ensuring that their medication management processes are as safe as possible, particularly in light of the unique issues that the older adult population may face.

Improving Medication Safety

Older adult patients face a number of factors that increase their patient safety risks: the aging process itself, the onset of potentially multiple chronic conditions, and polypharmacy. With medication use often a core aspect of caring for older adult patients, organizations need to ensure that their medication management processes, particularly in light of this particular population, work well to reduce the risk of unwanted ADEs. As identified, particular medication-related issues exist for older adult patients: polypharmacy, nonadherence to medicine regimens, and older adult-specific high-alert medication issues. Each of these issues presents particular medication safety challenges and opportunities for health care organizations. Improving on each of these issues can help reduce the chance of risks for older adult patients.

Staff Training and Orientation

Not all staff will have the same degree of experience in providing care for the special needs of older adult patients. Consider the following strategies when looking to improve staff training and education in relation to older adult patients:[11]

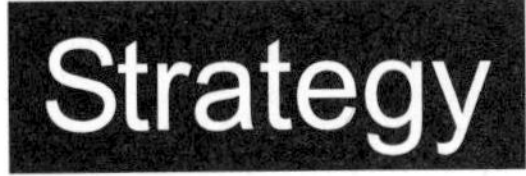

Multidisciplinary approaches. An older adult patient will often enter a health care organization with multiple conditions and health concerns, requiring input from a variety of professions, including nursing, pharmacy, physical therapy, and nutrition, to name a few. Ongoing care planning and assessment meetings between interdisciplinary teams of health care professionals can be an essential means for collaborating on the care of a patient and can help prevent any ADEs.

Strategy

Advanced care professionals. There is clearly a lack of gerontologically trained physicians, though many medical schools are now offering older adult–specific training for all medical students. Such specialists as gerontological nurse practitioners, elder care pharmacists, and clinical nurse specialists practicing as advanced practice nurses often have extensive knowledge and ability to assess and review the care of older adult patients to ensure that their needs are met.

Strategy

Orientation for new staff. In those settings where the organization may care for a variety of populations—such as in ambulatory, home care, or hospitals—it can be helpful to take time to orient staff to the particular concerns for older adult patients, particularly in relation to their medication use and any harmful interactions.

Strategy

Older adult medicine consultation. Some experts, such as older adult nursing experts Judith T. Rocchiccioli, Ph.D., R.N., professor of nursing at James Madison University, and Julie Sanford, D.N.S., R.N., associate professor of nursing at University of South Alabama, suggest establishing a comprehensive older adult medicine consultation service that could offer medication education to patients and even provide multidisciplinary team consultations. They suggest that the following evaluations could be part of the consultation:[12]

- Drug appropriateness or polypharmacy
- Psychosocial disposition
- Cognitive dysfunction or unmanageable behavior in patients with dementia

- Functional decline
- Falls risk
- Nutrition
- Urinary incontinence or catheter care
- Pressure ulcers
- Ethical issues

Medication Reconciliation

At the onset of care and in an ongoing manner, monitoring an older adult patient's medication use is essential. One study of home care patients found that 16% of patients had skipped a medication in the last 24 hours, 6% were taking the incorrect dose, and 5% were experiencing adverse effects from their medication.[12] Medication reconciliation is an important first step toward monitoring and managing the medication that an older adult patient takes. Many studies have indicated that prescribing providers are often unaware, or uninformed, about the medications that their patients are taking. In addition, many are unaware of the over-the-counter medicines or home-based remedies that a patient may take.[13]

In its rationale for its National Patient Safety Goal relating to medication reconciliation, The Joint Commission stresses that patients are at high risk for harm from ADEs when communication about medications is not clear. The rationale also states that the chance for communication errors can increase whenever there are changes in the individuals involved in a patient's care. Communicating about the medication list to ensure that it is accurate and reconciling any discrepancies whenever new medications are ordered or current medications are adjusted are essential to reducing the risk of transition-related adverse drug events.[14] The need for medication reconciliation is not simply necessary on admission to an organization but also important throughout the continuum of care for that patient. Any changes in medication should be documented, along with key aspects of medication use being communicated appropriately at times of discharge or transfer of care.

Working closely with the older adult patient to identify and monitor any and all medicines that the patient is taking is an important part of ensuring his or her safety. Consider the following steps in an older adult patient medication reconciliation strategy:[13]

- *"Brown bag" it.* Ask the patient to bring in (or provide, if the patient is in the home) all prescribed and non-prescribed medications and review them; this includes over-the-counter medications, herbs, and vitamins. Instruct the patient to check all areas in the home (for example, the kitchen, bathroom, and bedroom).
- *Screen.* Screen for adverse drug interactions. If these are identified, report to the prescribing provider the medications of concern.
- *Identify.* Identify the primary or secondary medical diagnosis related to each prescribed medication. If that is unknown, request the diagnosis from the prescribing provider.
- *Provide the list to the prescribing provider(s).* Provide the whole list (over-the-counter and prescribed) to the prescribing provider(s) and a list of corresponding diagnoses.
- *Verify.* Verify the prescribed medications and related diagnoses with the prescribing provider(s).
- *Provide a list to the patient.* Provide the medication list to the patient and/or caregiver. This list should also include the dose and frequency of these medications. Encourage the patient to share this list with the prescribing provider or other providers as needed. Instruct him or her to take the list every time he or she goes to a physician appointment.
- *Ensure that medication reconciliation is part of the discharge or transfer-of-care process.* When an older adult patient is discharged into home care or long term care from a hospital, for example, the hospital should provide a list of all medications the patient uses. This process should be clearly communicated to the patient and family as well.

Because he or she is the most consistent aspect of the medication reconciliation process, the patient has a crucial role to play. He or she cannot only be of great assistance to a health care organization in helping compile the medication reconciliation accurately upon admission to that organization, but he or she can also be educated and engaged in ensuring that any changes that need to be communicated are clearly documented.

Patient Education

Integral to any effective medication safety strategy is a patient education component. In the case of older adult patients and their often complex medication regimens, ensuring that patients are well educated, engaged in safety, and consistently following their prescribing provider's instructions is of the utmost importance. Consider the following strategies for building a robust and effective patient medication education program:

Strategy

Introduce an older adult patient medication education clinic. Because there are other education clinics to work with patients on managing their chronic illnesses (a diabetes clinic, for example), it could be helpful to also hold an older adult patient medication education clinic. This could be particularly effective in an ambulatory setting. A multidisciplinary approach could be effective as well, with elder care pharmacists participating, for example, to review medications for participating patients. The clinic could also provide specialized training and discussion for patients on medicines that are frequently prescribed for older adult patients or on the safe and unsafe interactions between prescribed medicines and, for example, over-the-counter medicines or herbs and certain foods. Organizations could pool resources and collaborate on such a clinic by working with other local organizations to host a community clinic.

Strategy

Don't wait until the day or time of discharge to provide patient education. A hospital or ambulatory surgical center stay can be a stressful and overwhelming experience for a patient and his or her family. Discharge by itself, with the education and instructions for aftercare and the anticipation of a time of recovery at home, admission into home care, or admission into a long term care facility, is no exception. To help a patient and family better understand what will happen after discharge, the organization should work with the patient on an ongoing basis to educate him or her on medication use and how to follow the prescriber's instructions. In addition, discharge education can be reinforced with a follow-up phone call from the organization.

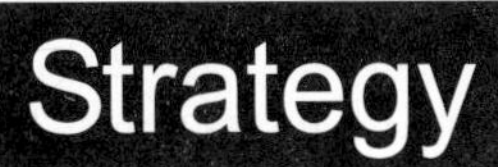

Provide older adult patients with multiple learning approaches. Do not rely on only one technique or approach to educate patients. Some patients, for example, may nod politely while in a consultation with a physician to indicate that they have understood what the doctor is saying, when in fact they may be confused but do not wish to interrupt or appear to criticize the doctor. A follow-up phone call or written instructions (written at a fifth-grade level and printed in a readable format) can help the patient review what was instructed during the doctor visit.

Strategy

Engage the patient in his or her own learning and patient safety. Don't hesitate to stress to the patient the importance of his or her active involvement in his or her own care. Provide him or her with ways to communicate with the organization if he or she has any concerns regarding medication safety. Remind him or her of his or her obligation to learn about and understand what his or her medications are for and how they should be taken. Reinforce the value of the patient contacting the organization if he or she has any concerns or confusion over his or her medications or if he or she notices any adverse effects. Brainstorm with the patient about ways to keep home medication safe (keeping medicines out of the sight of children) and to ensure his or her own safety (using pill boxes, calendars, or other electronic "reminders" to take medication).

Using Technology to Encourage Older Adult Medication Safety

Medication safety can be enhanced by the use of technology. With the use of the electronic medical record, computerized physician order entries (CPOE), automated dispensing machines, and smart pumps, to name a few, health care organizations can introduce consistency and systematization into their medication management processes, which can help reduce the incidence of medication-related adverse events. Table 3-3 represents a discussion of some potentially beneficial technologies that could help encourage older adult medication safety. It's important to note that these technologies can be used in organizationwide medication management and not just be limited to older adult patient medication safety.

Conclusion

Medication safety is crucial for any patient, regardless of age, special needs, or population. As such, organizations are charged to ensure that their overall medication management

Table 3-3. Common Medication Safety Technologies

Medication-Related Technology	Overview of Use
Using the computer for adverse drug event detection and alerts	Several studies have demonstrated the effectiveness of using computerized detection and alert systems to detect ADEs. Computerized ADE alert monitors use rule sets to search signals that suggest the presence of ADEs. The most frequently studied rule sets (or "triggers") are those that search for *drug names* (for example, naloxone, kayexalate), *drug-lab interactions* (for example, heparin and elevated PTT), or *lab levels alone* (for example, elevated digoxin levels) that frequently reflect an ADE. Simple versions can be implemented with pharmacy and laboratory data alone, although the yield and positive predictive value of signals is higher when the two databases are linked. Further refinements can include searches for International Classification of Diseases (ICD-9) codes and text searches of electronic nursing bedside charting notes or outpatient notes for *drug-symptom combinations* (for example, medication list includes an angiotensin converting enzyme inhibitor, and the patient notes mention "cough"). Although these refinements do increase the yield of monitors, they require linkage to administrative databases or electronic medical records. The information captured with computer monitors is used to alert a responsible clinician or pharmacist, who can then change therapy based on the issue in question. Systems are designed to alert the monitoring clinician in various ways. Alerts can go to one central location (for example, hospital pharmacist) or to individual physicians. Monitoring pharmacists typically review the alert and contact the appropriate physician if they determine that the alert has identified a true event. The alert modality also varies based on the available technology, from printed reports, to automatic paging of covering physicians, to display of alerts on computer systems (either results or ordering applications). It should be emphasized that computerized prescriber order entry is not a requirement for these monitors. Thus, a simple version of this approach could be implemented in most U.S. hospitals. Computerized real-time monitoring facilitates detection of actual and potential ADEs and notification of clinicians. This in turn may aid in the prevention of ADEs or decrease the chances that ADEs will cause harm. The monitors also yield improvements in secondary measures relating to the length of time until response and the quality of response.

Table 3-3. Common Medication Safety Technologies (Continued)

Medication-Related Technology	Overview of Use
Automated dispensing machines	Automated dispensing systems are drug storage devices or cabinets that electronically dispense medications in a controlled fashion and track medication use. Their principal advantage lies in permitting staff to obtain medications for inpatients at the point of use. Most systems require user identifiers and passwords, and internal electronic devices track nurses accessing the system, track the patients for whom medications are administered, and provide usage data to the hospital's financial office for the patients' bills. These automated dispensing systems can be stocked by centralized or decentralized pharmacies. Centralized pharmacies prepare and distribute medications from a central location within the hospital. Decentralized pharmacies reside on nursing units or wards, with a single decentralized pharmacy often serving several units or wards. These decentralized pharmacies usually receive their medication stock and supplies from the hospital's central pharmacy. More advanced systems provide additional information support aimed at enhancing patient safety through integration into other external systems, databases, and the Internet. Some models use machine-readable code for medication dispensing and administration. Automated dispensing devices have become increasingly common either to supplement or replace unit-dose distribution systems in an attempt to improve medication availability, increase the efficiency of drug dispensing and billing, and reduce errors. A 1999 national survey of drug, dispensing and administration practices indicated that 38% of responding hospitals used automated medication dispensing units and 8.2% used machine-readable coding with dispensing.[15] Three-fourths of respondents stated that their pharmacy was centralized, and of these centralized pharmacies, 77% were not automated. Hospitals with automated centralized pharmacies reported that more than 50% of their inpatient doses were dispensed via centralized automated systems. Half of all responding hospitals used a decentralized medication storage system. One-third of hospitals with automated storage and dispensing systems were linked to the pharmacy computer. Importantly, about half of the surveyed hospitals reported drug distributions that bypassed the pharmacy, including floor stock, borrowing patients' medications, and hidden drug supplies.

continued

Table 3-3. Common Medication Safety Technologies (Continued)

Medication-Related Technology	Overview of Use
Computerized prescriber order entry (CPOE)	The use of CPOE refers to a variety of computer-based systems of ordering medications, which share the common features of automating the medication ordering process. Basic CPOE ensures standardized, legible, complete orders by only accepting typed orders in a standard and complete format. At times, clinical decision support systems (CDSS) are implemented without CPOE. Isolated CDSSs can provide advice on drug selection, dosages, and duration. More refined CDSSs can incorporate patient-specific information (for example, recommending appropriate anticoagulation regimens) or incorporate pathogen-specific information, such as suggesting appropriate anti-infective regimens. After viewing such advice, the physician proceeds with a conventional handwritten medication order. Literature supports CPOE's beneficial effect in reducing the frequency of a range of medication errors, including serious errors with the potential for harm. Fewer data are available regarding the impact of CPOE on ADEs, with no study showing a significant decrease in actual patient harm. Similarly, isolated CDSSs appear to prevent a range of medication errors, but with few data describing reductions in ADEs or improvements in other clinical outcomes. Finally, the studied CDSSs address focused medication use (for example, antibiotic dosing) rather than more general aspects of medication use. Further research should be conducted to compare the various types of systems and to compare "home-grown" with commercially available systems. Such comparisons are particularly important because the institutions that have published CPOE outcomes have generally been those with strong institutional commitments to their systems. Whether less-committed institutions purchasing "off the shelf" systems will see benefits comparable to those enjoyed by "pioneers" with home-grown systems remains to be determined. Studying the benefits of such complex systems requires rigorous methodology and sufficient size to provide the power to study ADEs. Further research also needs to address optimal ways for institutions to acquire and implement computerized ordering systems.

Table 3-3. Common Medication Safety Technologies (Continued)

Medication-Related Technology	Overview of Use
Smart pumps	Infusion pumps with dose calculation software, sometimes referred to as "smart pumps," offer the opportunity to identify and correct pump-programming errors. Incorrectly programming intravenous pumps is one of the most common types of medication errors. When the error occurs with high-hazard drugs, it can result in serious ADEs, because there is little ability to correct the error before it reaches the patient. Smart pumps offer the capability for a hospital to preprogram its standard concentrations and to program upper and lower dose limits. When implemented well, the pump will alert the nurse if it has been programmed outside of safe limits and will prevent administration of doses that are considered by the hospital to be unsafe.[13] The Institute for Healthcare Improvement makes the following recommendations for the safe use of smart pumps: ■ Before deploying these pumps, standardize concentrations within the hospital. Asking the nurse to choose among several concentrations increases the risk of selection error. ■ Before deploying these pumps, standardize dosing units for a given drug (for example, agreeing to always dose nitroglycerin in terms of mcg/min or mcg/kg/min, but not both). Asking the nurse to choose among several dosing units increases the risk of selection error. ■ Before deploying these pumps, standardize drug nomenclature (for example, agreeing to always use the term KCl, but not Potassium chloride, K, Pot Chloride, or others). Asking the nurse to remember and choose among several possible drug names increases the risk of selection error. ■ Perform a Failure Modes and Effects Analysis on the deployment of these devices. ■ Ensure that the concentrations, dose units, and nomenclature used in the pump are consistent with those used on the medication administration record, the pharmacy computer system, and the electronic medical record. ■ Meet with all relevant clinicians to reach agreement on the proper upper and lower hard and soft dose limits. ■ Monitor overrides of alerts to assess if the alerts have been properly configured or if additional quality intervention is required. ■ Be sure the "smart" feature is used in all parts of the hospital. If the pump is set up volumetrically in the operating room, but the "smart" feature is used in the intensive care unit, an error may occur if the pump is not properly reprogrammed. ■ Be sure there are upper and lower dose limits for bolus doses, when applicable. ■ Engage the services of a human factors engineer to identify new opportunities for failure when the pumps are deployed. ■ Identify a procedure for the staff to follow in the event a drug must be given that is either not in the library or when its concentration is not standard. ■ Deploy the pump in all areas of the hospital. If a different pump is used on one floor and the patient is later transferred, this will create new opportunities for failure. Also, there may be incorrect assumptions about the technology available to a given floor or patient. ■ Consider using "smart" technology for syringe pumps as well as large volume infusion devices.

continued

Table 3-3. Common Medication Safety Technologies (Continued)

Medication-Related Technology	Overview of Use
Using telemedicine	Telemedicine is a relatively new technology that allows health care providers to work with and monitor patients remotely. This can include patient-provider communication, equipment monitoring, and communication (or the transmitting of information) between providers. This can be particularly useful for patients in remote settings, where access to health care services may be more limited. This form of technology can provide health care organizations with more effective access to older adult patients and could help monitor them for safety risks, such as falls, medicine use (or nonuse), or ongoing monitoring of wounds and other chronic ailments.
Source: *http://www.ahrq.gov*	

processes are focused not only on providing excellent quality of care but also on ensuring their safety. Older adult patients face special concerns in relation to medication safety, particularly due to the risks inherent in polypharmacy and an older adult patient's potential need for high-risk medications. Taking time to assess how well your organization's medication management system serves the needs of geriatric patients can help protect this vulnerable population and reduce the chance for adverse events. Chapter 4 looks at infection control and the special issues for organizations to consider in relation to older adult patients.

References

1. Col N., Fanale J.E., Kronholm P.: The role of medication noncompliance and adverse drug reactions in hospitalizations of the elderly. *Arch Intern Med* 150:841–845, 1990.
2. The Joint Commission: http://www.jointcommission.org/sentinelevents (accessed Mar. 21, 2009).
3. Mager D.: Medication errors and the home care patient. *Home Healthc Nurse* 25:152, Mar. 2007.
4. Grogan T., et al.: Keep your older patients out of medication trouble. *Nursing* 36(9):44–47, 2006.
5. Bergman-Evans B.: Evidence-based guideline: Improving medication management for older adult clients. *J Gerontol Nurs* pp. 6–13, Jul. 2006.
6. Sherman F.T.: Medicational nonadherence: A national epidemic among America's seniors. *Geriatrics* 62(4):5–6, Apr. 2007.
7. Snowden A.: Medication management in older adults: a critique of concordance. *Br J Nurs* 17(2):114–119, 2008.
8. Osterberg L., Blaschke T.: Adherence to medication. *N Engl J Med* 353:487–497, 2005.
9. Barber N., et al.: Patients' problems with new medication for chronic conditions. *Qual Saf Health Care* 13(3):172–175, 2004.
10. Jasniewski J.: Putting a lid on medication-related falls. *Nursing* 36(6):22, 2006.
11. Rocchiccioli J., et al.: Polymedicine and aging: Enhancing older adult care through advanced practitioners. *J Gerontol Nurs* pp. 19–24, Jul. 2007.
12. Ellenbecker C.H., et al.: Nurses observations and experiences of problems and adverse effects of medication management in home care. *Geriatr Nurs* 25(3):164–170, 2004.
13. Marek K.D., Antle L.: "Medication management of the community-dwelling older adult." In *Patient Safety and Quality: An Evidence-Based Handbook for Nurses.* AHRQ: http://www.ahrq.gov/qual/nurseshdbk/ (accessed Mar. 21, 2009).
14. The Joint Commission, National Patient Safety Goal, 08.01.01, http://www.jointcommission.org/NR/rdonlyres/31666E86-E7F4-423E-9BE8-F05BD1CB0AA8/0/HAP_NPSG.pdf (accessed Mar. 21, 2009).
15. Institute for Healthcare Improvement: http://www.ihi.org/IHI/Topics/PatientSafety/MedicationSystems/Changes/IndividualChanges/ImplementSmartInfusionPumps.htm (accessed Mar. 21, 2009).

Chapter 4

Infection Control Issues for Older Adults

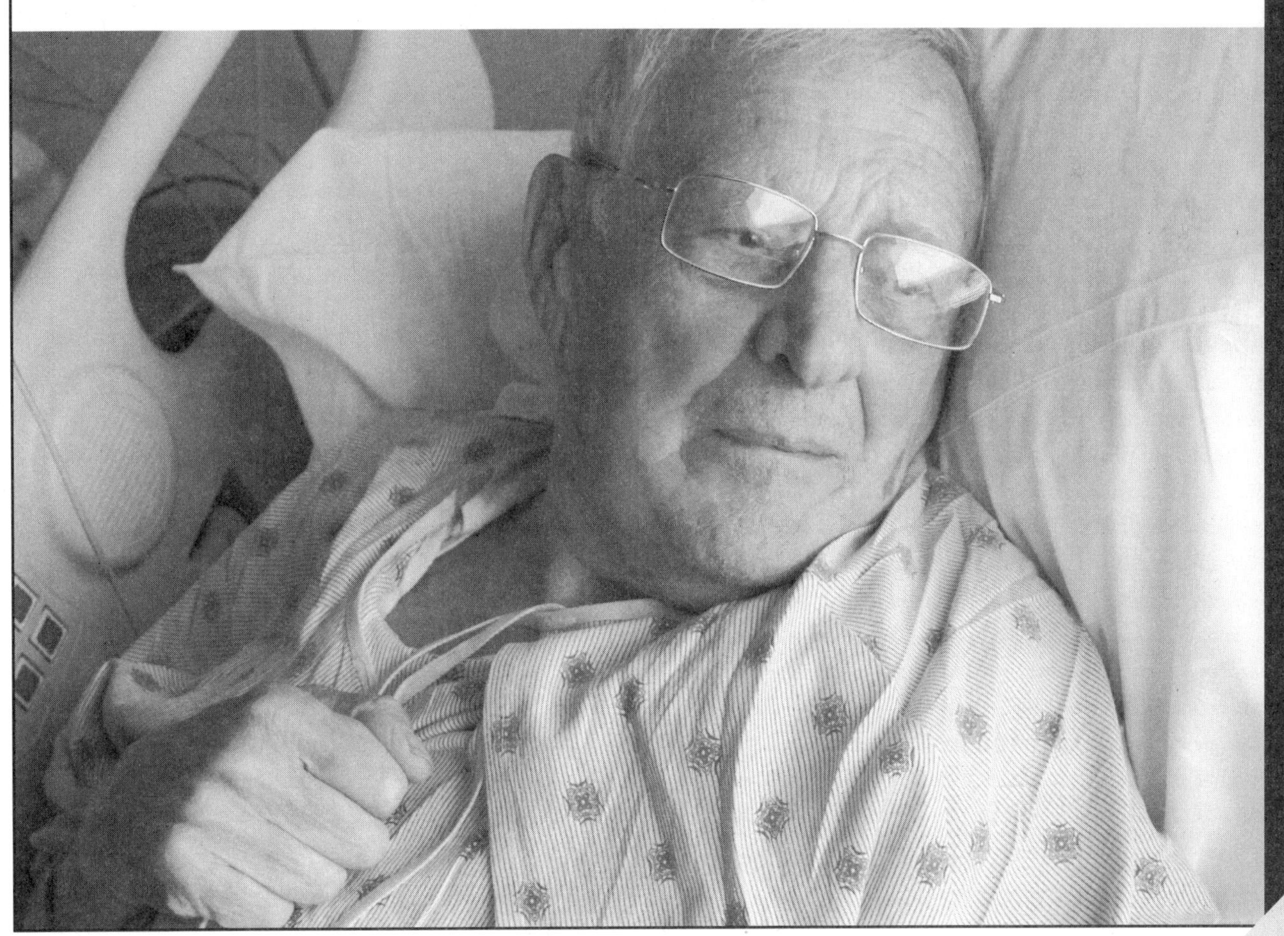

Along with medication management, infection control (IC) is a major patient safety issue for health care organizations. The Centers for Disease Control and Prevention (CDC) estimates that on an annual basis, nearly two million patients in the United States receive an infection in hospitals, and about 99,000 of these patients die as a result of their infection. The CDC also estimates that 32% of all health care–associated infections (HAIs) are urinary tract infections, 22% are surgical-site infections (SSIs), 15% are pneumonia (lung infections), and 14% arc bloodstream infections.[1] Infections are also a complication of care in other settings, including long term care facilities, home care, and ambulatory care settings. In the long term care setting alone, there are an estimated 1.6 to 3.8 million infections annually.[2] This health care crisis does not impact the United States alone, with countries such as the United Kingdom estimating that each year in England there are at least 300,000 cases of hospital-associated infection, causing about 5,000 deaths and costing their national health system as much as $1.5 billion in health care costs.[3] Globally, it is estimated that at any one time, more than 1.4 million people worldwide are suffering from infections acquired in hospitals.[4,5] HAIs occur worldwide and affect both developed and developing countries. In developed countries, between 5% and 10% of patients acquire one or more HAIs, and 15%–40% of patients admitted to critical care are thought to be affected.[6]

Older adult patients are more vulnerable to infections than their younger adult counterparts, with some estimates placing them at 3 times the mortality from pneumonia and 5 to 10 times from urinary tract infections. Older adult patients currently account for more than 15 million emergency department visits each year in the United States.[7] As a result of older adult patients' increased susceptibility to infection and their often vulnerable and frail health, an organization must work diligently to reduce the incidence of HAI and firmly establish good infection prevention methods. Approximately 1.5 million older adult patients reside in nursing homes, and it is estimated that anywhere from 3% to 15% acquire an infection in those facilities.[8] Experts also expect the incidence of infections in long term care facilities to increase as pathogens are becoming more resistant to antibiotic therapy.[9] This means that organizations could face an even more challenging time combating multidrug-resistant organisms (MDROs) and should be working to institute safe practices in relation to preventing and controlling infections.

Staff should know how to identify risk factors for infection in their older adult patient populations, and health care organizations should put systems in place to help prevent or reduce the incidence of HAIs. Older adult patients—many of whom might suffer from chronic illnesses, lack of mobility, and immunodeficiency—are especially vulnerable. Patients with indwelling devices, such as urinary, intravenous lines, or central venous catheters, and those undergoing invasive therapy, such as home infusion, ventilator support, and dialysis, are considered high-risk populations, as is anyone undergoing surgery or other invasive procedures.

In addition to providing education, organizations must communicate with all licensed independent practitioners, staff, students, and volunteers about their IC goals. People need to know their roles in preventing the spread of infection. Providing staff with concrete data of infection rates, educating them on ways to improve safety and reduce infections, having a robust patient education plan, and practicing diligent IC can go a long way toward ensuring compliance throughout the organization. Good venues for communicating such information to staff include in-services, newsletters, staff meetings, intranet sites, and breakroom bulletin boards.

Older Adult Patients and Infection Control

Recognizing the signs of infection on receiving a patient is one of the keys to IC as an organization. If a patient has an infection or has been exposed to one, an organization should be prepared to deal with it. Because older adult patients are more vulnerable to the effects of infection, reducing the incidence of infection in the organization can make a significant impact on older adult patient safety.

Effective initial assessments of older adult patients should include an IC assessment to determine if any infections are present and what, if any, interventions should be put in place. Some organizations have a robust IC department with dedicated infection prevention and control practitioners (ICPs). In those situations, ICPs can play an important role in assisting with any potential infection concerns or in helping develop the assessment tools that can identify any IC concerns, particularly in relation to the vulnerabilities faced by older adult patients. In settings where there is no dedicated IC staff, the responsibilities for IC will often fall to quality improvement staff. Overall, however, whether an organization has or does not have a dedicated IC staff on hand, all staff must be empowered to assess and respond to IC risks and issues.

Common Infections and Special Concerns for Older Adult Patients

Urinary Tract Infections

Urinary tract infections (UTIs) are common HAIs, accounting for approximately 40% of such infections in the United States alone. More than 80% of UTIs are associated with an indwelling urinary catheter, and risk increases with duration of catheterization. Geriatric age and urinary catheters can increase the risk for UTI.

Influenza and Pneumonia

Pneumonia is associated with high mortality rates, increased length of stay, and increased resource utilization. Pneumonia was recently found to be the leading cause of HAIs in medical/surgical intensive care units (ICUs), accounting for 31% of all hospital-onset infections. Risk factors for pneumonia include chronic pulmonary disease, severe underlying illness, older age, impaired airway reflexes, mechanical ventilation, and nasoenteric intubation.

Recent research indicates that in the United States, pneumonia is the fifth leading cause of death among older adult patients, with nursing home–associated pneumonia being associated with a 53% mortality rate.[7]

Although influenza impacts patients of all ages, it can have a particularly severe impact on older adult patients. Currently 90% of deaths related to influenza occur among older adult patients age 65 and over.[7] Effective influenza vaccination can help reduce the incidence of influenza among older adult patients. Joint Commission–accredited long term care organizations are now asked to comply with a National Patient Safety Goal that asks them to reduce the risk of influenza and pneumococcal disease in institutionalized older adults. It requires that long term care organizations do the following:

- Develop protocols to determine whether to administer the influenza vaccine to a resident.
- Implement protocols for residents identified as high risk for influenza.
- Develop and implement protocols for administering the pneumococcus vaccine.
- Develop and implement protocols to identify new cases of influenza and to manage outbreaks.

Catheter-Related Bloodstream Infections

Catheter-related bloodstream infections are less common than UTIs or pneumonia but can greatly affect outcomes and costs of care. Risk factors include age and the severity of underlying illness. Other common risk factors include errors in intravascular catheter insertion and management and low nurse-to-patient ratio.

Surgical-Site Infections

SSIs are a serious patient safety concern. The risk factors for SSIs include a contaminated, dirty, or infected wound; prolonged surgery; or a preoperative risk class greater than II, according to American Society of Anesthesiologists criteria.[10]

See Table 4-1 on page 50 for a list of the most common risk factors for SSIs.

The Basics: Emphasizing Infection Control Procedures and Educating Staff, Patients, and Family Members

Hand Hygiene

Hand hygiene is at the core of any effective IC process. Staff, patients, and family members should always be instructed to wash hands or use alcohol gel, as indicated. Depending on the organization, different interventions should be part of an organization's focus on infection prevention and control. The following section discusses some IC interventions and offers tips and strategies for implementation. The Joint Commission established a National Patient Safety Goal requiring accredited organizations to follow CDC or World Health Organization (WHO) hand-hygiene guidelines. *See* Sidebar 4-1 on page 51 for information on CDC and WHO guidelines.

Comprehensive hand hygiene is the most effective way to prevent the spread of infection. It is such a simple act, and yet many health care organizations have significant trouble achieving acceptable staff compliance rates. Staff are too busy or too distracted or do not value the importance of rigorous hand hygiene enough to engage in the activity as

Table 4-1. Surgical Site Infection Risk Factors After Cardiac Surgery[10]

Patient-Related:

- Preoperative ventilator use
- Chronic pulmonary disease
- Elevated body mass index
- Duration of ICU stay
- Diabetes mellitus
- Prior cardiac surgery
- American Society of Anesthesiologists score
- Advanced age
- Hospital admission greater than 48 hours before surgery

Procedure-Related:

- Coronary artery bypass graft valve surgery
- Duration of cardiopulmonary bypass
- Use of temporary pacing wires
- Perioperative blood transfusion
- Duration of surgery
- Bilateral mammary artery—unilateral mammary artery—saphenous vein graft
- Intraoperative aortic balloon pump use
- Postoperative resternotomy

Modifiable:

- Nasal carriage of *Staphylococcus aureus*
- Skin-shaving technique: razors, clippers
- Smoking
- Perioperative hyperglycemia

well as they should. Proper hand hygiene is a major component not only in breaking the chain of infection but also of an effective IC program. It is also a requirement of the National Patient Safety Goals. Organizations must implement CDC or WHO guidelines to ensure proper hand hygiene within the organization. How do organizations improve the hand-hygiene practices of their staff and work toward proper hand hygiene organizationwide? Following are a few suggestions.

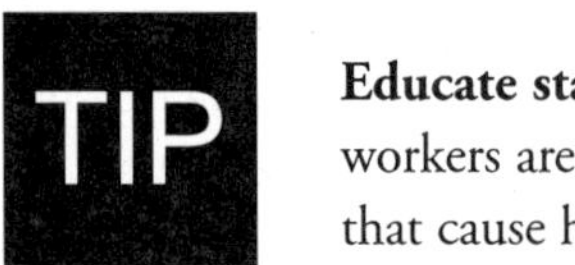

Educate staff. In some cases, health care workers are not aware of the activities that cause hand contamination. Although dressing an open wound would be an obvious activity following which most staff would wash their hands, some less obvious procedures, such as helping a caesarean patient to stand up and begin walking, might not be viewed as requiring hand hygiene. In addition, because there is a delay between improper hand hygiene and the emergence of an infection, many health care providers do not see the cause-and-effect relationship between thoroughly cleaning their hands and preventing infection. For staff to realize the importance of proper hand hygiene and engage in it at appropriate times, organizations should provide information on when hand hygiene is appropriate as well as real statistics that illustrate its importance. This information can be incorporated during staff in-services, on posters displayed in patient and breakrooms, or through company newsletters and e-bulletins.

Even if staff see value in hand hygiene, there might be some confusion as to when it is appropriate to use hand rubs versus hand washing. Organizations should educate staff on the appropriate times to wash their hands versus using an alcohol-based hand rub. For example, when hands are visibly dirty or contaminated with proteinaceous material or are visibly soiled with blood or other body fluids, staff should wash their hands with soap and water. If hands are not visibly soiled, staff can use soap and water or an alcohol-based hand rub for routinely decontaminating hands.

Create a culture that promotes hygiene. For staff to regularly comply with hand-hygiene procedures, an organization can and should foster a culture in which it is not only important to engage in hand hygiene, but it is completely unacceptable not to do so. This type of culture already exists in certain areas of health care. For example, no one should go into an operating room (OR) and touch the patient if he or she has not performed a preoperative hand preparation, and anyone in the OR can and should tell someone, even the chief of surgery, "I'm sorry, you didn't do your hand preparation, so you'll need to go out."

This culture tends to be absent in other settings, where staff usually feel reluctant to challenge those with more authority to comply with hygienic protocols. To achieve full hand-hygiene compliance, a culture of expectation must be reinforced by leadership. Several studies have shown that when administration makes overt and strong statements that hand hygiene is important, behavior does change. Organizations cannot expect overnight change, however, because behavioral changes are difficult to initiate and slow to take hold when you have to address existing mindsets and regularly give reminders of proper behavior.

To track changes in culture and identify areas for continued work, it might be helpful to periodically monitor hand-hygiene adherence and provide feedback to personnel about their performance. Monitoring the volume of alcohol-based hand rub used per 1,000 patient days is one way of monitoring hand-hygiene practice. Another way is conducting observational studies of hand-washing practices and hand-rub use.

Make hand hygiene convenient. Where high volume is a major factor in noncompliance, an organization should think about what products it currently provides for hand hygiene. For example, introducing alcohol-based hand rubs can make hygiene procedures quicker and more effective and may increase overall

Sidebar 4-1. CDC and WHO Hand Hygiene Guidelines

CDC Hand-Hygiene Guidelines

In late 2002, the Centers for Disease Control and Prevention (CDC) released some specific guidelines regarding the washing of hands in health care institutions, including hospitals, clinics, and nonhospital environments, such as dialysis centers. These guidelines acknowledge that hand hygiene is a critical component of patient safety and can really save lives in health care settings. They also note that health care providers are not traditionally supportive of hand-hygiene regimens and offer some solutions to help improve compliance, such as the appropriate use of alcohol-based hand rubs.

For the CDC's full report on hand hygiene, go to http://www.cdc.gov/mmwr/PDF/rr/rr5116.pdf.

WHO Hand-Hygiene Guidelines

In 2006, the World Health Organization (WHO) also released an advanced draft of hand-hygiene guidelines for health care organizations worldwide titled *WHO Guidelines on Hand Hygiene in Health Care*. It includes a thorough review of evidence on hand hygiene in health care and specific recommendations on how to improve practices and reduce transmission of pathogenic microorganisms to patients and health care workers.

For access to the WHO's advanced draft of its guidelines, go to http://www.who.int/patientsafety/information_centre/Last_April_versionHH_Guidelines%5B3%5D.pdf.

Note: *As of this printing, the WHO guidelines are noted as being an "advanced draft." The WHO notes that a final version will be published on the http://www.who.int Web site soon. Organizations should check there for the most up-to-date version of the guidelines.*

Crosswalk of Guidelines with Joint Commission Hand Hygiene National Patient Safety Goal

The Joint Commission has established a National Patient Safety Goal requirement that states that all ambulatory care, behavioral health care, critical access hospitals, home care, hospitals, laboratories, long term care, and office-based surgeries should comply with current WHO guidelines or CDC guidelines. To help organizations compare the two guidelines, a crosswalk of the guidelines was published in the February 2008 issue of *Joint Commission Perspectives®*.

hand-hygiene compliance. Organizations can make an alcohol-based hand rub available inside the entrance to the patient's room or at the bedside, in other convenient locations, and in individual pocket-sized containers to be carried by caregivers.

Enlist clinical leader support. Clinical leaders, whether physicians, nurses, or informal leaders, set the tone for other caregivers. Seeing these people perform hand washing or hand antisepsis on a regular basis encourages other professionals to follow suit and feel more comfortable speaking up when they notice someone else neglecting such protocols.

Encourage patient involvement. In addition to training staff, it is important for patients to realize their role in proper staff hand hygiene. Organizations should provide education to patients about their role and encourage patients and families to ask their health care providers whether they have washed their hands. Some organizations provide all staff with buttons that say, "Ask me if I've washed my hands." Sometimes, this simple question from a patient can help a provider remember this important infection-prevention strategy.

Do not rely on gloves. Although gloves play an important role in preventing the spread of infection, the use of gloves is not a substitute for good hand hygiene. Gloves might have tiny perforations that allow pathogens to reach the skin, or staff might forget to remove gloves after touching a patient and before entering another area. Bacteria can be spread from one part of the body to another if staff do not replace soiled gloves between tasks. Used gloves should also be removed before staff touch such surfaces as door handles or telephones. Staff should be educated on when gloves are appropriate, and hand washing or hand antisepsis should be carried out before and after contact with every patient, whether or not gloves are used.

Special Infection Control Concerns for Older Adult Patients

- ***Masks for respiratory diseases.*** To prevent the transmission of infectious disease, staff, patients, and family should be encouraged to wear masks because it is a proven IC strategy. Researchers have found that those adults who wore masks while in their homes were four times more likely than nonwearers to be protected against respiratory viruses, including the common cold.[11]

- ***Isolating patients.*** When an organization makes the decision to isolate a patient, it might involve placing the patient in a private room; requiring visitors and health care workers to wear protective apparel, such as gowns, gloves, and masks; and restricting the movement of the patient outside the room. In some cases, visitors are restricted to limit the spread of the infection.

  Within an emergency management plan, organizations should identify how they will isolate large numbers of patients and make sure those patients receive prompt, safe, and documented care.

  In addition, organizations should have a system in place to manage how such supplies as linens, eating utensils, and clothing are provided and managed for isolated patients. Organizations should have an emergency supply source in place before an influx of sick patients arrives. One way for hospitals to do so is to examine their current inventories of supplies, bedding, food, and water for natural disasters. When preparing for a biological or chemical attack, looking at those inventories and determining what needs to be added would be a logical starting point.

- ***Use precautions.*** Standard precautions should be used for patients at all times. Considering the risks that older adult patients face, staff should be encouraged to use the precautions as much as possible. *See* Sidebar 4-2 on page 53 for guidelines on standard precautions.

- ***Personal protective equipment (PPE).*** Staff, patients, family, and visitors may need additional IC protection by using such things as PPE to carry out standard precautions. This PPE includes gowns, masks, and eye protection and face shield (if splashes or sprays of blood or body fluids are likely). The reasons for the use of PPE should be clearly communicated to the family and the patient.

Sidebar 4-2. Standard Precautions

Standard precautions are the basic level of IC that should be used in the care of all patients all the time.

- Use standard precautions in the care of all patients to reduce the risk of transmission of microorganisms from both recognized and nonrecognized sources of infection.
- Applies to blood, all body fluids, secretions, and excretions (except sweat) whether or not they contain visible blood; nonintact skin; and mucous membranes.
- Personal protective equipment (PPE) to carry out standard precautions includes:
  - Gowns
  - Masks
  - Eye protection and face shield (if splashes or sprays of blood or body fluids are likely)
- **Hand hygiene**—always—following any patient contact
  - Wash hands for 20 seconds with soap and warm water, especially if visibly soiled. Clean hands with alcohol-based hand rub if not visibly soiled.
- **Gloves**
  - Use clean, nonsterile gloves when touching or coming into contact with blood, body fluids, secretions, or excretions
  - Apply gloves just before touching mucous membranes or contacting blood, body fluids, secretions, or excretions
  - Remove gloves promptly after use and discard before touching non-contaminated items or environmental surfaces and before providing care to another patient
  - Wash hands immediately after removing gloves
- **Gowns**
  - Fluid resistant, nonsterile
  - Protect soiling of clothing during activities that may generate splashes or sprays of blood, body fluids, secretions, and excretions
  - Apply gown before performing such activities
- **Mask, face shield, eye protection**
  - Protect eyes, nose, mouth, and mucous membranes from exposure to sprays or splashes of blood, body fluids, secretions, and excretions
  - Apply appropriate protection before performing such activities
    - Masks and respirators
    - Other face and eye protection
- **Patient Care Equipment**
  - Avoid contamination of clothing and the transfer of microorganisms to other patients, surfaces, and environments
  - Clean, disinfect, or reprocess nondisposable equipment before reuse with another patient
  - Discard single-use items properly

Monitoring Special Infections

Health Care–Associated Infections

With American hospitals estimated as experiencing 1.7 million HAIs and approximately 99,000 deaths each year, and part of the United Kingdom, England, estimating 300,000 HAIs resulting in 5,000 deaths annually, the need for preventing and reducing the incidence of HAIs is urgent.[1,3] Although these statistics are by themselves quite serious, the more disturbing fact is that many of these infections are potentially preventable. Although it is true that some people who acquire infections in a health care organization are frail or immunocompromised, there are also healthy people who enter health care organizations for elective procedures, expecting to go home in good health, and instead acquire infections that sometimes result in death. Unfortunately, infections pose a significant threat to patient safety, and organizations must work to prevent them when possible and mitigate their effects when prevention cannot be accomplished.

In addition to the safety risks associated with infections, HAIs are extremely costly to health care organizations. A recent report estimates that the efforts to treat these infections add nearly $17 billion to health care costs every year.[12] A recent study in the *Journal of the American Medical Association* noted that selected infections due to medical care result in an average length of stay (LOS) increase of nearly 10 days, excess charges of more than $38,000, and an increase in patient mortality of nearly 5%.[13] Reacting to infections is much more costly than preventing them, and, in the current health care environment where every expense must be defended, the large price tag of reacting to infections instead of preventing them is indefensible.

Possible Infection Control Measures for the Prevention of Transmission of *Clostridium difficile*

Barrier precautions

- Gloves
- Gown
- Hand washing
- Isolation

Environmental cleaning

- Rooms
- Toilets
- Single-use rectal thermometers

Other strategies

- Antibiotic restriction
- Metronidazole for asymptomatic carriers

Traditionally, the spotlight of concern surrounding HAIs has shone predominantly on hospitals, but that has now changed. With shorter LOS following inpatient treatment and the movement of certain types of invasive procedures to outpatient settings, greater focus moves to infections associated with other health care settings, including the home. Organizations of all types must address a variety of different infections, including the following:

- Catheter-associated UTIs
- Bloodstream infections—often associated with intravascular devices
- Community and health care–associated pneumonia
- Skin and soft tissue infections
- SSIs

The many reasons that infections occur in a health care setting including the following:

- Inadequate hand hygiene
- Transmission of MDROs
- Inadequate staffing levels
- Sick or immunocompromised patients
- Technically sophisticated and invasive interventions that present new opportunities for infection

See the box above for information on measures to prevent the transmission of *Clostridium difficile.*

Surgical-Site Infections

SSIs account for 14% to 16% of all HAIs among hospitalized patients.[14] Many studies have identified that the incidence of SSIs contribute to lengthier stays in the hospital and increased costs. The Institute for Healthcare Improvement's Web site notes that an estimated 2.6% of nearly 30 million operations are complicated by SSIs each year.[15]

According to the CDC's National Healthcare Safety Network that monitors reported trends in nosocomial infections in participating U.S. acute care hospitals:

- 38% of all nosocomial infections in surgical patients are SSIs
- 4% to 16% of all nosocomial infections among all hospitalized patients are SSIs
- 2% to 5% of operated patients will develop SSIs
- SSI increases LOS in hospital by an average of 7.5 days
- $130 million to $845 million per year are the estimated national costs in the United States[1]

According to the Institute for Healthcare Improvement, ideal perioperative care has four key components: appropriate use of antibiotics, appropriate hair removal, perioperative glucose control (major cardiac surgery patients cared for in an ICU), and perioperative normothermia (colorectal surgery patients). (**Note:** *The last two components of care are supported by clinical trials and experimental evidence in the specified populations. They may prove valuable for other surgical patients as well.*)

Device-Related Infections

Certain devices commonly used in the health care settings have been linked to a higher risk of causing infection due to the invasive nature of these devices and their use. The kinds of device-related infections include the following:

- Intravascular catheter-related bloodstream infection
- Catheter-related UTI
- Ventilator-associated pneumonia
- Dialysis-related infections

These infections are not only costly to deal with but can exact a high cost to patient safety. The CDC estimates that of the 1.7 million HAIs each year in the United States alone, 32% are UTIs and 14% are bloodstream infections, comprising two of the most common four HAIs reported. In addition, it estimates that globally there are 1.4 million patients with HAIs at any time, including device-related infections.

For a copy of the CDC's 2002 Guidelines for the Prevention of Intravascular Catheter-Related Infections, go to http://www.cdc.gov/mmwr/PDF/rr/rr5110.pdf.

Conclusion

IC can impact an entire organization and all the patients for which it cares. Older adult patients are particularly vulnerable to infection, and its adverse impact can constitute a high percentage of those adversely impacted by HAIs and community-associated infections. Organizations need to ensure that, as with all systems and processes to provide high-quality safe care, their IC processes accommodate any special concerns for older adult patients. The following chapter explores the issue of falls and falls prevention among geriatric patients.

References

1. Centers for Disease Control and Prevention: *Estimates of Healthcare-Associated Infections.* http://www.cdc.gov/ncidod/dhqp/hai.html (accessed Mar. 21, 2009).
2. Strausburgh L.J., Joseph C.L.: The burden of infection in long-term care. *Infect Control Hosp Epidemiol* 21:674–679, 2000.
3. House of Commons Committee of Public Accounts: *Improving Patient Care by Reducing the Risk of Hospital-Acquired Infection: A Progress Report.* http://www.publications.parliament.uk/pa/cm200405/cmselect/cmpubacc/554/554.pdf (accessed Mar. 21, 2009).
4. Tikhomirov E.: WHO Programme for the control of hospital infections. *Chemioterapia* 3:148–151, 1987.
5. Vincent J.L.: Nosocomial infections in adult intensive care units. *Lancet* 361:2068–2077, 2003.
6. Lazzari S., Allegranzi B., Concia E.: Making hospitals safer: The need for a global strategy for infection control in healthcare settings. *World Hosp Health Serv* pp. 32, 34, 36–42, 2004.
7. Caterino J.M.: Evaluation and management of geriatric infections in the emergency department. *Emerg Med Clin North Am* 26:319–343, 2008.
8. Mody L.: Infection control issues in older adults. *Clin Geriatr Med* 23:499–514, 2007.
9. Crogan N., Evans B.: *Clostridium difficile*: An emerging epidemic in nursing homes. *Geriatr Nurs* 28(3):161–164, 2007.
10. Hospital-Onset Infections: A Patient Safety Issue, http://www.annals.org/cgi/content/full/137/8/665 (accessed Feb. 19, 2009).
11. Med India: *Face Masks Could Boost Protection Against Respiratory Illnesses.* http://www.medindia.net/news/Face-Masks-Could-Boost-Protection-Against-Respiratory-Illnesses-46816-1.htm (accessed Feb. 19, 2009).
12. Bhutta A., et al.: Reduction of bloodstream infections associated with catheters in paediatric intensive care unit: stepwise approach. *BMJ.* 334:362–365, 2007.
13. Zhan C., Miller M.: Excess length of stay, charges and mortality attributable to medical injuries during hospitalization. *JAMA* 290:1868–1874, Oct. 15, 2003.
14. Emori T.G., Gaynes R.P.: An overview of nosocomial infections, including the role of the microbiology laboratory. *Clin Microbiol Rev* 6(4):428–442, 1993.
15. Institute for Healthcare Improvement: http://www.ihi.org/ihi/Topics/PatientSafety/SurgicalSiteInfections/SurgicalSiteInfectionsCaseForImprovement (accessed Mar. 21, 2009).

Chapter 5

Fall Prevention and Older Adults

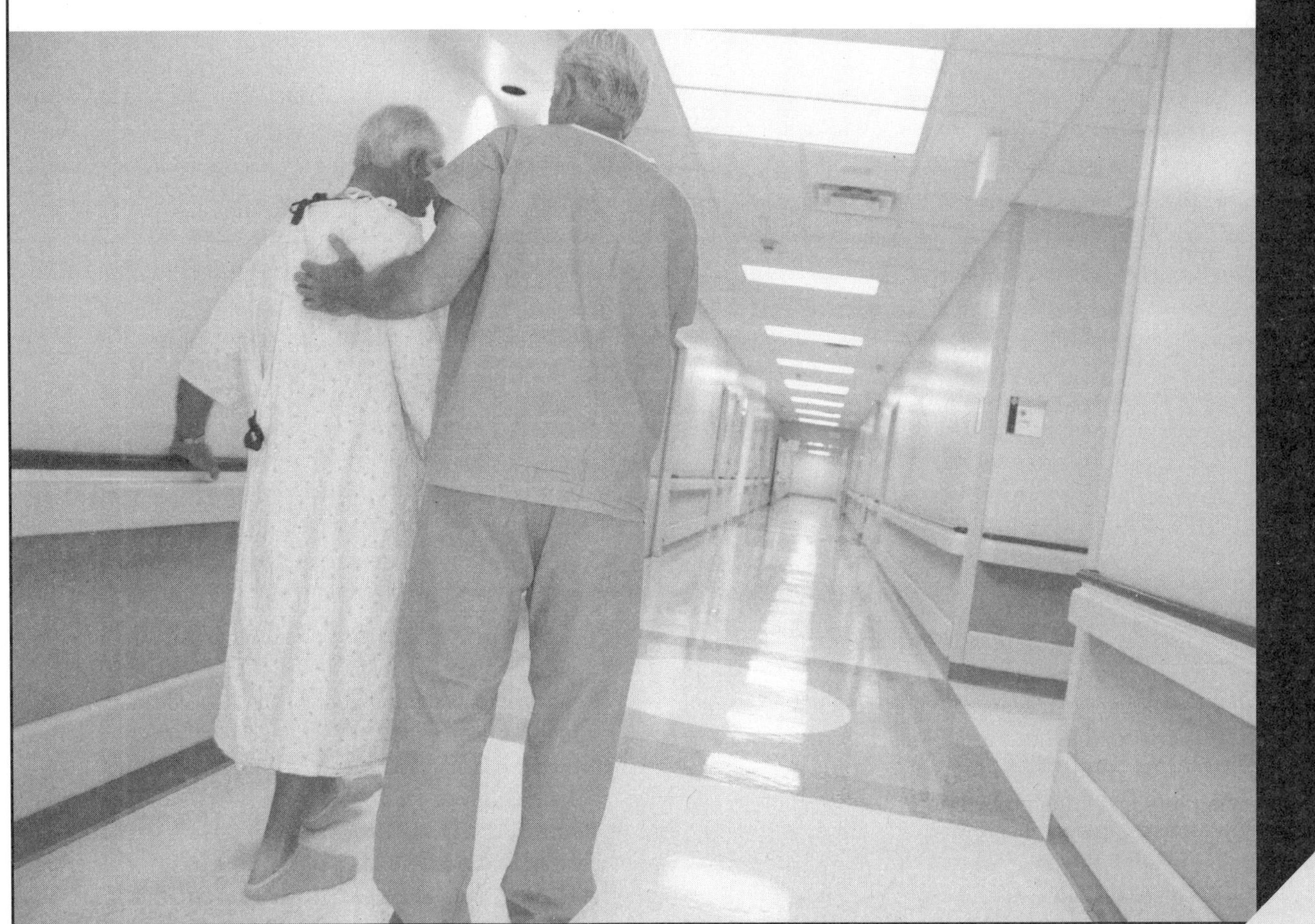

On October 1, 2008, the Centers for Medicare & Medicaid Services (CMS) stopped reimbursing hospitals for the treatment of certain "conditions that could reasonably have been prevented," including falls.[1] Falls, along with seven other conditions (including pressure ulcers, surgical-site infection, and objects being inadvertently left in after surgery), were selected by CMS to be on this list of the so-called "never events," "because they greatly complicate the treatment of the illness or injury that caused the hospitalization."[2]

The World Health Organization estimates that 28% to 35% of people globally age 65 and over fall each year, with that number increasing to 32% to 42% for those over 70 years of age.[3] According to the Centers for Disease Control and Prevention, in the United States in 2004, approximately 15,000 older adult patients died from injuries related to unintentional falls, and 1.8 million older adult patients were treated in emergency departments for nonfatal injuries from falls. More than 400,000 of those patients were hospitalized.[4]

Roughly 250,000 nursing home residents in the United States suffer a serious fall injury on an annual basis, with estimated costs of $4.9 billion in 2005.[5] International estimates approximate that 30% to 50% of long term care residents fall each year, and 40% of them experienced recurrent falls.[3] Studies undertaken in Sweden, the United States, and the United Kingdom have drawn attention to the significant direct health care costs required for the treatment of fall-related injuries. Two recent studies have used aggregated data to examine the current and projected costs of fall injuries in Australia. One study examined all injury categories and found that fall injuries were the most costly of any injury mechanism. The second study, undertaken on behalf of the Australian government, found that aging of the Australian population in the next 50 years will have a significant impact on the health system due to the increased number of older people suffering fall-related injuries. The study concluded that prevention strategies will need to deliver a reduction in falls incidence of approximately 66% in order to maintain cost parity with current health system costs.[6]

Falls and their resulting harm to patients have long been considered unwelcome and alarming events for a patient, his or her family, and the health care organization. Falls can happen in any setting and can result in serious injury and even death. Often synonymous with the high risks of aging, falls are certainly not exclusively in the realm of older adult patients, but they do happen most frequently in that population. Long recognized as a major patient safety crisis, recent U.S. data point to 41 fall-related deaths per 100,000 population.[7] Falls are the sixth-leading cause of death among older adult patients.[8]

Falls and fall-related injuries are defined in the following ways:

- *Falls:* An unplanned descent to the floor (or extension of the floor, for example, trash can or other equipment) with or without injury. All types of falls are included, whether they result from physiological reasons or environmental reasons.[7]
- *Fall-related injuries:*[7]
    - *None* indicates that the patient did not sustain an injury secondary to the fall
    - *Minor* indicates those injuries requiring a simple intervention
    - *Moderate* indicates injuries requiring sutures or splints
    - *Major* injuries are those that require surgery, casting, and further examination
    - *Deaths* refer to those that result from injuries sustained

The goal of a health care organization should be to reduce the incidence of falls among patients. This chapter focuses on the risk factors that go into falls, approaches to fall-risk assessments, falls prevention strategies, staff training, and patient education.

In the Notes from the Field on page 59, Elaine Buccellato shares some insight and guidance for organizations hoping to improve their falls prevention and reduction efforts.

Evaluating Fall Risks

Older adult patients face many risk factors for falls and fall-related injuries. These risk factors need to be identified and understood so that organizations can plan for the particular risks and work to reduce the incidence of adverse events. A recent study on falls noted that older adult patients are more vulnerable to falls in the following ways:[9]

Notes from the Field: Improving Falls Prevention and Reduction

Elaine Buccellato, B.S.N., M.S., Joint Commission surveyor in the long term care and hospital settings, notes that falls prevention is a vital part of older adult patient safety. It is known that falls are a common occurrence for the elderly and a required quality measure for most health care organizations. Effective prevention strategies can mitigate the number of falls, but, more important, they can lessen the number and severity of injuries from falls. Health care organizations are required to have a falls prevention program in place. However, it is essential that the program is evaluated to ascertain whether it is working and achieving its goals.

Buccellato also points out the need for adequate resources and communication in relation to reducing falls. "For example, one nursing home's improvement plan was to have fall risk residents wear 'slip-free' socks at bedtime so that they would not slip as they got up to go to the bathroom at night. Some staff were aware of this new requirement, but the significance of this was not communicated clearly to all staff. At first, adequate supplies of the socks were on the linen cart, but they became less available. When there were not enough 'slip-free' socks on the linen cart, and the staff thought that the residents would be fine with regular socks, a workaround was created, and 'slip-free' socks were not used consistently. The number of falls increased. However, if the organization had monitored the new requirement to use 'slip-free' socks, until the practice was imbedded into the care routine, they would have noticed the lack of resources and that the staff was not complying with the new requirement."

"So, instead of reacting to the falls," Buccellato stresses, "organizations should put their focus and effort on the inputs to the fall prevention process and really assess if the new requirement is being implemented consistently. This illustrates the benefits of Robust Performance Improvement, which stresses the importance of watching the 'inputs to an improvement plan as well as the outcomes.'" Buccellato emphasizes that an improvement process should always be well planned, have little variation, and be clearly communicated to the staff who have a role to play in the new "safer" process.

- Muscle weakness for older adult patients increased fall risk four-fold
- Balance deficits and history of falls increased fall risk three-fold
- Cognitive impairment, age greater than 80 years, and visual impairment increased risk three-fold
- Gait deficits and depression doubled the risk

These additional risk factors that have been identified:

- Neurological disease
- Demographics, such as age, ethnic background, housebound status, and living alone
- Use of assistive devices, such as a cane or walker
- Environmental hazards, such as rugs, distance to the call button, being alone in the bathroom (after a surgery, and so on)
- Poor nutrition
- Impaired activities of daily living
- Multiple medications (polypharmacy)
- Hypotension
- Poor score on the Get-Up-and-Go test (patient unable to stand up from a sitting position)
- Special toileting needs (urinary incontinence and frequency, altered elimination)

Medications can pose a significant risk for falls in older adult patients. Studies have found that certain medications have been linked to an increased falls risk, due to side effects or their effect on the patient:[10]

- Sedatives
- Psychotropics
- Analgesics
- Cardiovascular agents
- Antidepressants
- Antihypertensives
- Anticoagulants
- Anticonvulsants
- Anticholinergics/bladder relaxants
- Antipsychotics

Medications can increase the risk of falling in a number of ways, most commonly:

- Sedation
- Impaired balance and reaction time
- Orthostatic hypotension
- Drug-induced Parkinsonism

Sidebar 5-1. Examples of Fall Risk Factors

- A history of falls
- Fear of falling, causing a patient to restrict his or her own activity
- Illness, disease, or condition that impacts mobility or balance (such as coronary artery disease, dementia, tinnitus, strokes, or obesity)
- Multiple medication use (polypharmacy)
- Use of certain types of medication (such as high-risk medications like sedatives or beta blockers)
- Postural hypotension, a blood pressure drop from rising from the chair or bed, causing light headiness or giddiness
- Depression
- Glaucoma and cataracts (wearing bifocal glasses can distort vision when looking up and down)
- Cognitive impairment, dementia, or confusion
- Incontinence or frequency (getting up during the night can increase risk of falling)
- Inadequate diet, poor nutrition, all impacting muscle and bone strength
- Insomnia/poor sleep hygiene (patient is not alert to hazards in the environment)
- Alcohol (could lead to impaired judgment and also can react with a range of prescribed drugs, such as benzodiazepines)
- Weak muscles and joints/poor mobility and balance
- Gait deficit, impairment, or instability or use of an assistive device from such conditions as arthritis, foot problems, surgery, damage to inner ear, and neurodegenerative disorders
- Inappropriate clothing (long or trailing nightgowns or robes) or poorly fitted shoes or slippers
- Environmental hazards (such as rugs, slippery floors, or no grab rails or adaptations)[11]

As noted, polypharmacy can increase the chance of falls. With patients on multiple drug therapies, the chance of drug interactions or fall risk increases. *See* Chapter 3 for more information on medications that can impact falls.

From an environmental standpoint, the conditions of floors and bed and toilet height can be contributing factors to higher risk for falls among older adult patients. In addition, poor lighting and signage, clutter in rooms, and an inability to reach the call button are also risk factors for falls. *See* Chapter 2 for more discussion on the environment and falls, but consider the following tips in relation to fall reduction in the environment:[10]

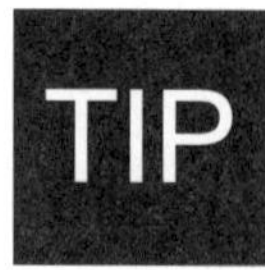

Keep beds in a low position with wheels locked for those patients identified as being at high risk.

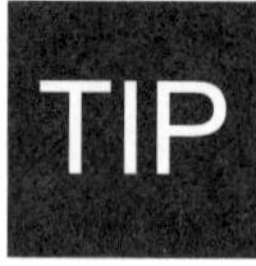

Relocate patients at high risk for falls closer to the nurses' station for ease of access by staff.

Ensure that the at-risk patient's bed is located as closely as possible to the bathroom.

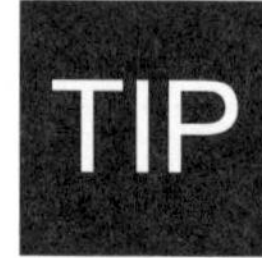

For high-risk patients, consider mandating that staff accompany patients to the bathroom.

Keep personal items and call buttons within easy reach.

Ensure adequate lighting is available.

Table 5-1. Risk Factors for Falls, Injuries, and Fall-Related Deaths

Intrinsic Risk Factors	Fall Risk	Injury Risk	Mortality Risk
Demographics			
• Age: Older Age (especially >70 yrs)	Yes	Yes	Yes
• Gender	Female	Female	Male > age 85
• Race	Caucasian	Caucasian	Caucasian
Cognitive Function			
• Cognitive impairment	Yes	No data	No data
• Fallophobia (fear of falling)	Yes	Yes	No data
• Inability to follow instructions	Yes	No data	No data
• Inability to adapt to changing environment	Yes	No data	No data
Physical Function			
• Gait problems	Yes	No data	No data
• Impaired ability to perform activities of daily living	Yes	Yes	No data
• Impaired muscle strength or range of motion	Yes	Yes	No data
• Poor/fair self-reported health	Yes	Yes	No data
• Roscow-Breslau impairment (functional status assessment)	No data	Yes	No data
• Vision problems	Yes	No data	No data
Physical Status			
• Body Mass Index (BMI) less than 22.8 kg/m2	No data	Yes	Yes
• Frailty	No data	Yes	Yes
• Low body weight (<58 kg=BMI 23 if height 5'3")	Yes	Yes	No data
Comorbidities			
• Alzheimer's disease	Yes	No data	No data
• Anemia (including mild anemia)	Yes	No data	No data
• Diabetes	Yes	No data	No data
• Diabetic foot ulcer	Yes	No data	No data
• Fall in the past 12 months	Yes	Yes	No data
• Parkinson's disease	Yes	No data	No data
• Postural hypotension	Yes	No data	No data
• Previous fracture	No data	Yes	No data
• Stroke	Yes	Yes	No data
• Subdural hematoma (chronic)	Yes	Yes	No data
• Syncope	Yes	No data	No data
• Vitamin D deficiency	Yes	Yes	No data
• Vitamin D deficient with low creatine clearance	Yes	No data	No data

continued

Table 5-1. Risk Factors for Falls, Injuries, and Fall-Related Deaths (Continued)

Intrinsic Risk Factors	Fall Risk	Injury Risk	Mortality Risk
Medications			
• Use of four or more medications	Yes	No data	No data
• Antiepileptics	No data	Yes	No data
• Antihypertensives	Yes	No data	No data
• Antiplatelet therapy	No data	No data	Yes
• Psychotropics	Yes	No data	No data
• Sedatives and hypnotics	Yes	No data	No data

Extrinsic Risk Factors	Fall Risk	Injury Risk	Mortality Risk
• Environmental hazards	Yes	No data	No data
• Footwear, nonsupportive (for example, slippers)	Yes	No data	No data
• Hospitalization, recent	Yes	No data	No data
• Wheelchair use, reckless wheelchair use	Yes	No data	No data

Source: *Currie, Leanne, Ph.D., R.N.: Fall and injury prevention.* Patient Safety and Quality: An Evidence-Based Handbook for Nurses. *AHRQ Publication No. 08-0043. Agency for Healthcare Research and Quality, Rockville, MD. http://www.ahrq.gov/qual/nurseshdbk/ (accessed Mar. 22, 2009).*

Consider treating floors with slip-prevention treatments.

Ensure adequate equipment is available to help patients move safely.

Sidebar 5-1 on page 60 and Tables 5-1, above, and 5-2, pages 63–64, provide examples of risk factors facing older adult patients for falls in the different settings.

Being able to predict the risks of and thereby work toward reducing the number of falls will help an organization achieve an important patient safety goal. Organizations have available a number of fall risk assessment tools to use, including the Hendrich II Fall Risk Model™, which was developed by Ann Hendrich, M.S.N., R.N., F.A.A.N., to assess a patient's risk for falling. It has been designed for use in the acute care setting, but its evidence-based principles of assessment can be applied in other settings as well. Table 5-3, page 65, is an example of the Hendrich II Fall Risk Model. For more information, go to http://www.ahincorp.com.

Organizations may also find it preferable and advisable to devise their own assessment tool based on evidenced-based findings of risk factors and their own organization-driven data relating to falls and fall risk. The risks identified in Tables 5-1 and 5-2 could lay a good foundation, depending on the health care setting and its particular needs in relation to older adult patients.

Strategies to Prevent or Reduce Falls Risk

Preventing falls risk is a significant responsibility for health care organizations. The prevention of falls is so

Table 5-2. Risk Factors for Falls and Injuries in Acute and Long Term Care

Intrinsic Risk Factors	Fall Risk	Injury Risk
Demographics		
• Age	Across ages	Older
• Gender	Male	Female
Cognitive Function		
• Agitation	Yes	Yes
• Anxiety	Yes	No data
• Cognitive impairment	Yes	No data
• Impulsivity	Yes	No data
• Inability to follow instructions	Yes	No data
• Short-term memory loss	Yes	No data
Physical Function		
• Fall history	Yes	Yes
• Fatigue	Yes	No data
• Gait problems	Yes	No data
• Impaired muscle strength	Yes	No data
• Impaired physical functioning	Yes	No data
• Toileting needs increased	Yes	No data
• Postural hypotension	Yes	No data
• Visual impairment	Yes	No data
Physiologic Status		
• Alkaline phosphatise level elevated	Yes	No data
• Anemia	Yes	No data
• Parathyroid hormone deficiency	Yes	Yes
• Prolonged bleeding time	No data	Yes
• Vitamin D deficiency	Yes	Yes
Comorbidities		
• Alzheimer's disease	Yes	No data
• Depression	Yes	No data
• Diabetes	Yes	No data
• Comorbidities in general	Yes	No data
• Multiple sclerosis	Yes	No data
• Parkinson's disease	Yes	No data
• Stroke	Yes	No data
• Syncope	Yes	No data

continued

Table 5-2. Risk Factors for Falls and Injuries in Acute and Long Term Care (Continued)

Intrinsic Risk Factors	Fall Risk	Injury Risk
Medications		
• Anticoagulants	No data	Yes
• Antiepileptics	Yes	No data
• Chemotherapeutics	Yes	No data
• Laxatives	Yes	No data
• Psychotropics	Yes	No data
• Sedatives and hypnotics	Yes	No data

Extrinsic Risk Factors	Fall Risk	Injury Risk
Other Factors		
• Staffing	Yes	No data
• Time of day	Yes	No data
• Electroconvulsive therapy (in behavioral health)	Yes	No data
• Being physically challenged (in rehabilitation)	Yes	No data

Source: *Currie, Leanne, Ph.D., R.N.: Fall and injury prevention.* Patient Safety and Quality: An Evidence-Based Handbook for Nurses. *AHRQ Publication No. 08-0043. Agency for Healthcare Research and Quality, Rockville, MD. http://www.ahrq.gov/qual/nurseshdbk/ (accessed Mar. 22, 2009).*

important that Joint Commission and Joint Commission International–accredited health care organizations are asked to meet a National Patient Safety Goal requesting them to implement a falls prevention program with the express aim of reducing the incidence of falls.

Experts have long stressed the importance of putting into place effective strategies to reduce fall risks. The following are some general suggestions for intervention. Table 5-4, page 66, includes some evidence-based recommendations for screening and assessment for falls in a variety of settings. Table 5-5, page 67, and Table 5-6, page 68, include some evidence-based interventions in the community (Table 5-5) and acute care and long term care settings (Table 5-6), respectively.

Consider the following strategies for preventing or reducing the risk of falls.

Multidisciplinary and Multifactorial Approach

Effective fall prevention requires input and participation from a wide array of disciplines. Preventing falls requires vigilance and attention, not simply from the nurse at the bedside, but from all staff who interact with a patient. This approach also requires that patients and families remain attentive to any changes or vulnerabilities that the patients may be experiencing. Recent research has indicated that those organizations that are seeing success in their fall prevention work have used multifactorial and multidisciplinary approaches.[12] Falls prevention is not merely achieved by having a low-height bed, for example. It is achieved by using a multitude of approaches, including the following:

- Assessing and reassessing by multiple staff in an ongoing manner
- Improving balance and exercise programs
- Advanced training and education of staff

Table 5-3. Hendrich II Fall Risk Model™

Risk Factor	Definition	Points	Score
Confusion Disorientation Impulsivity		4	
Symptomatic depression		2	
Altered elimination		1	
Dizziness Vertigo Sway Path Loss of balance		1	
Gender		1	
Any prescribed antiepileptics		2	
Any prescribed benzodiazepines		1	
Get Up & Go Test			
Ability to rise in a single movement		0	
Pushes up, successful in one attempt		1	
Multiple attempts, but successful		3	
Unable to rise without assistance during test (OR if a medical order states the same and/or complete bed rest is in order) * If unable to assess, document this on the patient chart with the date and time		4	
A score of 5 or greater = High Risk		TOTAL SCORE	

Source: *Copyright 2007 AHI of Indiana, Inc., all rights reserved, United States Patent #7,282.031. Used with permission.*

- Using technology to monitor a patient
- Patient education and empowerment
- Volunteer or staff companion
- Using hip protectors
- Using nonslip footwear
- Using low-height beds
- Patient access (or assistance) to the bathroom
- Medication assessment for risk factors
- Creating visual triggers for staff to know there is a high fall-risk patient
- Environmental aids or adaptive equipment to assist patients (call buttons, mobility aids, bedside cushions)

Effective falls prevention requires a multifaceted approach. For example, one organization's study found that although using an incident reporting system was a helpful way to learn about the types, causes, and frequency of patient falls, it was not sufficient as a sole source of data, because there was underreporting to the system. It found that a combination of the incident reporting system with a falls evaluation service provided more robust data.[13]

Table 5-4. Recommendations for Screening and Assessment

Evidence-Based Practice Recommendations	Research Implications
Community	
■ Screen all patients over age 65 during routine or other visit. ■ For patients who screen positive, refer to fall-injury prevention clinic for focused fall-injury risk assessment, if available. ■ Use a standardized risk assessment tool, such as Tinetti's nine-item screening tool for: 1. Mobility 2. Morale 3. Mental status 4. Distance vision 5. Hearing 6. Postural blood pressure 7. Back examination 8. Medications 9. Ability to perform activities of daily living.(**Note:** *This tool does not overtly assess for injury risk.*) ■ For patients older than age 65 years old who present to the emergency department with a fall, refer to primary care provider for focused fall-injury risk assessment.	■ Examine risk factors related to space and gender. ■ Identify barriers to widespread screening. ■ Examine barriers to establishing fall-injury prevention clinics. ■ Validate risk assessment instruments across culture, race, and language. ■ Examine predictive validity of injury risk factors, such as antiplatelet therapy, bleeding disorders, Vitamin D deficiency, and chronic subdural hematomas. ■ Develop instruments for patient self-assessment for fall and injury risk. ■ Examine the effect of identification in the emergency department using large, multicenter randomized controlled trials. ■ Identify barriers to widespread adoption.
Home Care and Long Term Care	
■ Screen patients of all ages. ■ Use a standardized risk assessment tool, such as Tinetti's nine-item screening tool (see above). ■ Reassess at regular intervals.	■ Validate home care assessment instruments. ■ Examine predictive validity of long term care minimum data set. ■ Examine best timing for reassessment in home care and long term care.
Acute Care Setting	
■ Screen patients of all ages. ■ Use a standardized risk assessment instrument, such as the Morse, Hendrich II, or Stratify tools. (**Note:** *These tools do not assess for injury risk.*) ■ Assess for injury risk for patients with injury risk factors, such as low body mass index, frailty, osteoporosis, Vitamin D deficiency, and antiplatelet therapy. ■ Reassess patients at regular intervals.	■ Develop and validate instruments for subgroups. ■ Validate instruments in multiple settings. ■ Explore predictive validity of physiologic factors, such as low creatine clearance, Vitamin D deficiency, and anemia. ■ Validate instruments that assess for injury risk. ■ Examine the best timing for reassessment.

Source: *Currie, Leanne, Ph.D., R.N.: Fall and injury prevention.* Patient Safety and Quality: An Evidence-Based Handbook for Nurses. *AHRQ Publication No. 08-0043. Agency for Healthcare Research and Quality, Rockville, MD. http://www.ahrq.gov/qual/nurseshdbk/ (accessed Mar. 22, 2009).*

Table 5-5. Recommendation for Community Setting

Evidence-Based Practice Recommendations	Research Implications
Fall Prevention	
■ Provide balance training with leg strengthening, such as tai chi. ■ Monitor medication side effects for patients older than age 65. ■ Limit medications to fewer than four, if possible. ■ Monitor and treat calcium and Vitamin D deficiency. ■ Manage underlying disorders, such as cardiac-related syncope, diabetes, and vision problems (for example, cataracts). ■ Provide home safety modifications. ■ Educate about use of thin-soled shoes (not running shoes). ■ Provide education about how to manage risky situations.	■ Examine effect of starting balance training at younger age (that is, 50 years). ■ Examine barriers to establishing and using balance training centers. ■ Identify medications with minimal side effect profiles for patients older than age 65. ■ Examine medication dosing for groups of medications. ■ Examine factors related to calcium and Vitamin D metabolism in relation to muscle function. ■ Explore factors to manage groups of disorders. ■ Explore other diseases that may predict falls. ■ Explore barriers to home safety modification. ■ Further explore shoe type for specific patient groups. ■ Explore fall prevention self-management strategies.
Injury Prevention	
■ Monitor for calcium and Vitamin D deficiency; provide supplements for fracture prevention. ■ Increase screening for patients on anticoagulant therapy, those with bleeding disorders, and for the frail and advanced in age. ■ Use bisphosphonates for patients with documented osteoporosis.	■ Conduct large studies that control for comorbidities, age, and other factors to explore efficacy of hip protectors in the community. ■ Identify safety measures for bleeding-injury prevention. ■ Explore interventions for those advanced in age and frail. ■ Explore safety of long-term use of bisphosphonates.

Source: *Currie, Leanne, Ph.D., R.N.: Fall and injury prevention.* Patient Safety and Quality: An Evidence-Based Handbook for Nurses. *AHRQ Publication No. 08-0043. Agency for Healthcare Research and Quality, Rockville, MD. http://www.ahrq.gov/qual/nurseshdbk/ (accessed Mar. 22, 2009).*

Table 5-6. Recommendations for Acute and Long Term Care

Evidence-Based Practice Recommendations	Research Implications
Fall Prevention	
■ Educate staff about safety. ■ Train medical team, including students and residents, for fall-injury risk assessment and post-fall assessment. ■ Use alarm devices. ■ Monitor medication side effects and adjust as needed. ■ Adjust environment (for example, design rooms to promote safe patient movement). ■ Provide exercise interventions (for example, tai chi) for long term care patients. ■ Provide toileting regimen for confused patients (for example, check patients every 2 hours). ■ Monitor and treat calcium and Vitamin D levels for long term care patients. ■ Treat underlying disorders, such as syncope, diabetes, and anemia.	■ Examine impact of safety education across interdisciplinary team. ■ Examine impact of alarms on caregiver satisfaction. ■ Examine effect of computerized decision support for medication management. ■ Examine cost effectiveness of environmental adjustments. ■ Examine usefulness of exercise interventions for acute care patients. ■ Study barriers to maintaining and sustaining monitoring activities. ■ Examine effects of calcium and Vitamin D management for acute care patients. ■ Examine constellations of disorders that might precipitate falls.
Injury Prevention	
■ Limit restraint use. ■ Lower bedrails. ■ In addition to fall rates, monitor injury rates. ■ Use hip protectors for older adults and long term care. ■ Use floor mats. ■ Monitor prothrombin time, international normalized ration (PT/INR) for patients at risk for falling. ■ Ensure post-fall assessment. ■ Use bisphosphonates for patients with documented osteoporosis.	■ Identify methods to overcome barriers to restraint reduction. ■ Study efficacy of environmental changes. ■ Establish fatal fall rates across settings. ■ Identify methods to overcome barriers to using hip protectors. ■ Examine effect of safety flooring. ■ Identify safety measures for bleeding-injury prevention. ■ Examine barriers to post-fall assessment. ■ Explore safety of long term use of bisphosphonates.

Source: *Currie, Leanne, Ph.D., R.N.: Fall and injury prevention.* Patient Safety and Quality: An Evidence-Based Handbook for Nurses. *AHRQ Publication No. 08-0043. Agency for Healthcare Research and Quality, Rockville, MD. http://www.ahrq.gov/qual/nurseshdbk/ (accessed Mar. 22, 2009).*

Table 5-7. Summary of Results Table—Post-Fall Assessment Algorithm

Grade of nurse completing form	Staff nurse 10	Sister/charge nurse 4	Clinical team leader 0	Other 1
All parts of form filled in correctly	Yes 12	No 0	Incomplete 3	
Outcome of assessment by nurse	No injury 8	Minor injury 7	Major 0	
Outcome of assessment by physician	No injury 11	Minor injury 4	Major 0	
Physician's attendance	Immediate 0	Same day 12 (2 not specified)	Next day (night) 1	
Category of physician's attendance appropriate	Yes 13	No 0 (2 not specified)		

Source: *Fenton W.: Introducing a post-fall assessment algorithm into a community rehabilitation hospital for older adults.* Nurs Older People *20:36–39 Dec. 2008. RCN Publishing Company, London. Used with permission.*

At England's South Birmingham Primary Care Trust, a community rehabilitation hospital for older adults, normal practice in the assessment of patients following a fall was often varied, because nurses did not assess patients in a standard manner and usually contacted a physician immediately, regardless of whether the patient was injured.

A small study was undertaken to develop an assessment tool to guide nurses in evaluation of older adult patients in community hospitals after a fall and to help them prioritize when a physician should be consulted—either immediately, the same day, or the next day. It was believed this would promote better use of resources and facilitate better communication between the nursing staff and physicians.[14]

Within the scope of the study, a multidisciplinary focus group of eight members, including a physiotherapist and an occupational therapist, selected for their interest and expertise in falls assessment and treatment met six times over 3 months. The group agreed with the concept of a preliminary toe-to-toe assessment by a registered nurse before the patient is moved with the inclusion of a body diagram to document injury sites.[14]

The refined tool became known as the "Post-Fall Assessment Algorithm," and the group coined the phrase "assess, look, feel" as a memory aide. The group felt the tool should be simple and concise, so that a nurse not trained in first aid would be confident to use it (*see* Table 5-7, above, and Figure 5-1, page 70).

Figure 5-1. Post-Fall Assessment Algorithm

Affix Patient ID label

Prelimary assessment prior to moving the patient. ASSESS, LOOK, FEEL (ALF)

1. Conscious → No → Check airway, breathing, circulation, initiate BLS procedure, immediate attendance
   ↓ Yes

2. Bleeding → Yes → Assess, stop bleeding → doctor
   ↓ No

3. Any bleeding from back of head → Yes → Call doctor (feel back of head), skull depression/swelling, loss of fluid from nostrils/ears
   ↓ No

4. FACE/HEAD
   Any cuts/bruises/swelling/broken glasses → Yes → Call doctor – if suspected fracture
   ↓ No

5. New pain → Yes → Call doctor – if suspected fracture
   ↓ No

6. NECK
   Any neck pain/bruising → Yes → Call doctor and immobilize neck with two pillows either side if suspected fracture
   ↓ No

7. TRUNK
   Any new pain → Yes → Call doctor
   ↓ No

8. UPPER LIMBS
   ASSESS, LOOK, FEEL and compare left and right → Yes → Call doctor and immobilize limb if suspected fracture or dislocation. Any swelling/deformities/new pain/loss of movement
   ↓ No

9. LOWER LIMBS
   ASSESS, LOOK, FEEL and compare left and right → Yes → Call doctor and immobilize limb if suspected fracture in the position you find them using pillows/rolled up blankets. Any external/internal rotation/shortening/swelling/loss of movement. Unable to bear weight—new problem
   ↓ No

1. Record pulse/blood pressure Yes No
2. Record neuro observations if head involved Yes No
3. Record location and type of injury on diagram
4. Record in medical notes and insert this form in medical notes
5. Doctor to be contacted in daytime hours to inform of fall/discuss injuries and urgency of attendence. Senior nurse to be contacted out of hours to be informed of fall/discuss injuries/urgency of doctor attendance. Please tick box:

Immediate attendence required ❑
Same day ❑
Next day ❑

Name:.................... (Print)
Signature:
....
Date: ....
Time: ....

If patient has sustained an injury, please inform matron/senior nurse.

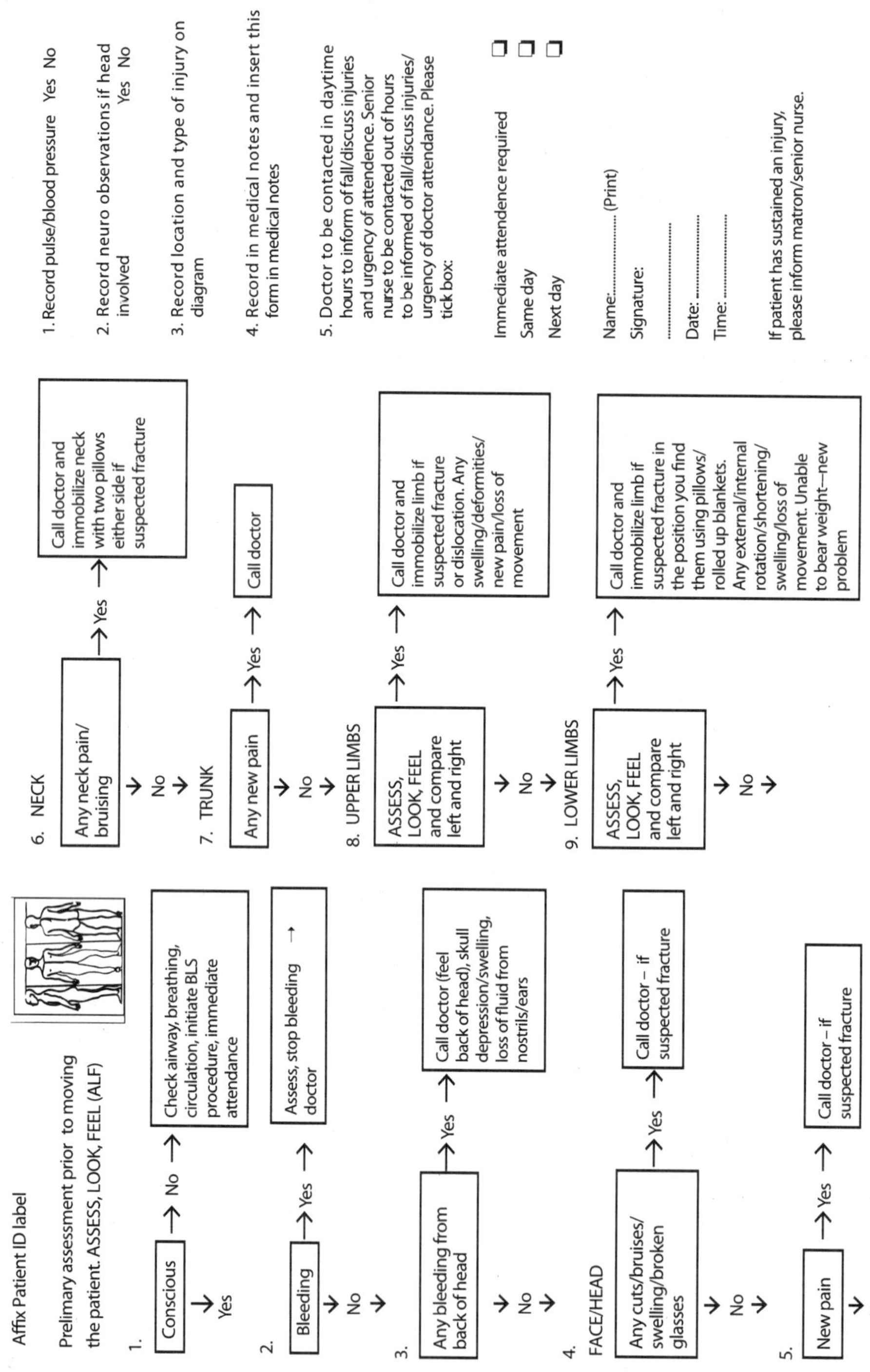

Figure 5-1 is a sample of the post-fall assessment algorithm.

Source: *Fenton W.: Introducing a post-fall assessment algorithm into a community rehabilitation hospital for older adults.* Nurs Older People *20:36–39, Dec. 2008. RCN Publishing Company, London. Used with permission.*

The Post-Fall Assessment Algorithm could be used by staff in other clinical areas for patients who have fallen, according to researchers. Staff required only brief training in the algorithm's use and found it a useful prompt. The researchers found the algorithm improves decision making regarding requesting attendance of a physician. Training in the use of the algorithm should form part of the overall falls awareness training, in the context of closing the loop between risk assessment, implementation of a multifactorial falls prevention plan, and assessment of injury should the patient fall.[14]

Frontline staff, such as nurses, certified nurses' assistants, physical/occupational therapy, nutritional staff, transport staff, and housekeeping staff, can be alert to any fall-risk concerns over a patient; health care providers can monitor a patient's risk factors to determine what risk may exist; organizations can put in place technological and environmental tools or aids to help the patient remain safe; specialized areas, such as pharmacy, physical/occupational therapy, and nutrition, can give input into a fall risk assessment tool. It is important to note that many organizations that have seen improvements in falls prevention state that having a multifaceted approach can be beneficial to the success of a program. Because falls are such a pervasive problem, it may be necessary to cover as many possibilities as possible.

An important component of any approach to reducing the incidence of falls among patients is having a consistent, organizationwide approach. The responsibility for driving an organizationwide commitment to reducing falls rests on leadership's shoulders. If leadership firmly states their engagement in reducing falls, it can empower staff to feel connected to the goal and help an organization achieve its broader patient safety goals. The fact is that more often than not when an organization (with its leadership) commits wholeheartedly to reducing a challenging patient safety problem, such as falls risk, then that organization is embracing the concept of a culture of safety.

Volunteer Companions

Some organizations have begun using volunteers to sit with a high fall-risk older adult patient to help monitor him or her in an ongoing manner for falls. One study in Australia had volunteers working during prime-time hours (8 A.M.–8 P.M.) to help monitor high-risk older adult patients on a older adult–specific unit. The hospital placed high-risk patients in an observation room, and volunteers worked in pairs, with one canvassing the unit for any wandering patients and the other sitting in the observation room with the patients. This study found that while volunteers were with patients, there were no falls among observed patients. Unfortunately, it did find that falls did take place in the observation room during nonvolunteer hours (the evening and overnight). It also found that during the study's time frame (over a 4-month period), 13 of the 45 volunteers recruited to sit with patients left the program.[15]

The volunteer system can have positive effects with a dramatic improvement in reducing risks for patient falls. But it appears resource intensive, and researchers note that its biggest strength lies in when the companion is with the patient. If organizations do not provide a multifaceted approach to monitoring patients, such as another means of observing patients while volunteers are not present or available, falls will still take place.

Consider the description offered in Table 5-8 on page 72 for the role of a volunteer companion.

Fall Monitors and Observation Approaches

Falls can take place at any time and in a variety of locations in a health care organization. For patients in a home care program, falls can take place anywhere in the home. Some organizations have begun using technology in different ways to try to them monitor and observe patients at risk for falls to help reduce the incidence of falls. In other cases, some have rearranged the geography of their unit or work area to accommodate improved approaches to observing high fall-risk patients. Consider the following approaches in your planning strategies:

Strategy

Video monitor. These video monitors link to cameras in patient areas where patients have been deemed to be at high risk for falls. Viewable in a specific location on a unit or floor (but out of the view of family and visitors to the area), staff can rotate time observing patients on a single unit or floor from a central location. This can allow for constant monitoring and help staff respond to potential falls. See the case study on pages 73–75 for one organization's positive experience with the use of video monitors to reduce falls.

Table 5-8. Description of the Volunteer Companion Role

Role Description	■ The volunteer companion is an unpaid member of staff, whose primary function is to observe those patients at high risk of falling.
Purpose of Role	■ Observe patients at high risk of falling and notify nursing staff of all potential occasions where the patients may fall. ■ Engage patient in social interaction and perform diversion activities as appropriate. ■ Complement the roles of paid staff, thereby enhancing service provision.
Activities	■ Observe patients in the allocated patient bay and intervene as required to minimize the risk of patients falling. ■ Recognize and immediately report any change in patients' behavior that could increase the risk of harming themselves or others. ■ Social interaction with patients is encouraged. ■ Perform diversional activities, including reading to patients, reminiscence, singing. ■ Perform recreational activities, including taking patients for a walk in the wheelchair. ■ Perform helping activities, including pouring a drink, cutting up food. ■ Perform therapeutic activities (for example, hand massage).
Activities Not to Be Performed	■ "Catching" a patient who is falling ■ Patient feeding ■ Patient transfer (from bed to chair/wheelchair) ■ Patient toileting
Responsibilities	■ Undertake the volunteer companion orientation and training program. ■ Volunteer for one 4-hour shift each week for the duration of the trial. ■ Ensure that all patient information is treated confidentially. ■ Respect the values, spiritual beliefs of patients. ■ Demonstrate sensitivity to privacy and dignity aspects of patient care. ■ The volunteer is covered by the hospital's workers compensation policy.
Reporting	■ The volunteers report to the hospital volunteer coordinator but work under the direct supervision of the registered nurse. ■ Nursing staff communicate relevant patient information at the commencement of the shift.
Remuneration	■ Nil, including no payment of expenses (for example, mileage reimbursement or travel expenses)

Source: *Giles L.C., et al.: Can volunteer companions prevent falls among inpatients? A feasibility study using a pre-post comparative design.* BMC Geriatr *6:11 2006. http://www.biomedcentral.com/1471-2318/6/11 (last accessed Mar. 22, 2009). Public domain.*

CASE STUDY

Spotlight on Improvement: Poudre Valley Hospital and Falls Reduction

Like all hospitals around the country, PVH has been looking for an effective approach to fall prevention in its patients. "Reducing falls has been a priority for PVH for years," explains Ric Deflesen, R.N., patient safety officer. "Earlier approaches to reducing falls began approximately 6 or 7 years ago. We studied the research, started a process improvement team, and shared and communicated best practices with staff, but we were not seeing a significant improvement."

PVH's initial improvement work was carefully thought out and creative. "We brought together our expertise and looked at a variety of interventions, everything from using a detailed assessment form to physical features, such as putting red dots on the door frame to indicate falls risk," says Deflesen.

But PVH could see that its interventions, while good ideas and effective to some extent, were not helping the falls rate decrease significantly. "We eventually changed the team to a monthly committee, because we realized that making improvements is multifactorial and requires an ongoing effort," Deflesen notes.

Redesigning the System

Assessments

PVH did not stop with changing its performance improvement team into a monthly committee. It redesigned its assessment form to more effectively designate those patients at high risk, established a mandatory requirement for bathroom accompaniment for high-risk patients, and introduced video monitoring on its neurosciences unit.

"Identifying high-risk patients is a crucial step toward reducing falls, so we implemented a process to assess high risk," Deflesen explains. He also notes that the previous assessment form, though well conceptualized, was less effective, because staff were tempted to make a subjective judgment regarding the patient's fall level and then document only symptoms that supported that level, overlooking those symptoms that might support a higher-risk level. PVH redesigned its assessment process to relieve staff from relying on their "pet symptom" when assessing for risk and instead look at the assessment form to guide the establishment of risk.

Deflesen notes that PVH has designed and implemented its own assessment form (*see* Figure 5-2, page 74). He explains that this was important because each organization faces its own challenges. "You have to know how falls happen in your area and ask the right questions that are relevant to you and your patients," he stresses. Now, with what they feel is a more simplified form, staff have been able to use it with less variation.

Bathroom Accompaniments

Probably one of the more striking elements of PVH's falls prevention program is its determination that no high-risk patient may go to the bathroom unaccompanied, a policy that PVH has had in place since September 2006. "We have a clear mandate: Someone has to be in the bathroom with the high-risk patient," Deflesen explains. It is not enough for a staff member to even be elsewhere in the room as there is a group of patients at risk for falling in the bathroom, requiring staff to be within reach of the patient. This was an adjustment for some staff and patients. For staff there was the concern over privacy and resource usage and for patient's privacy, factored in along with a concern over "bothering" the nurse. "But our mindset has been that

At-a-Glance

About the hospital: Poudre Valley Hospital (PVH) is a 241-bed hospital located in Fort Collins, Colorado, which provides such services as neurosciences, cardiology, trauma, orthopedics, bariatric services, cancer treatment, and women's and family care.

About the improvement: PVH instituted the following:

- An effective, concise falls-risk assessment for use by staff
- A process for staff to always accompany high fall-risk patients to the bathroom
- Enhanced video monitoring with select populations to help observe and prevent falls risk

Figure 5-2. PVH Falls Assessment Screens

☐ Any of these high-risk symptoms: Recent history of falls; balance or gait impairment/weakness or dizziness; cognitive impairment; orthostatic hypotension; bowel or bladder incontinence or frequency/urgency; unwillingness or inability to call for help

☑ Any of these moderate-risk symptoms: Use of environmental support for ambulation; communication or sensory deficit; alcohol or drug withdrawal, or potential for; sedative, hypnotic, tranquilizer, analgesic-naïve; laxatives or diuretics; hypotensive

☐ Any of these low-risk symptoms: Emotional upset, low morale, altered sleep patterns

Based upon your assessment above the following interventio [Moderate Risk]

High Risk Interventions	Moderate Risk Interventions	Low Risk Intervention
➢ Red magnet on door jam ➢ Siderails x 4 ➢ Low bed position ➢ Bed alarm ➢ Every 30 minute checks ➢ Call light within reach ➢ Remove obstacles ➢ Encourage toileting q 1-2 hours (attended in bathroom at all times) ➢ Gait belt or up with assist when walking/standing ➢ Assess for use of Stedy device ➢ Adjust lighting as appropriate ➢ Use glasses/hearing aids as appropriate	➢ Side rails x 2 or 4 ➢ Low bed position ➢ Every hour checks ➢ Call light within reach ➢ Remove obstacles ➢ Offer toilet every 1-2 hours ➢ Assess for use of Stedy device ➢ Adjust lighting as appropriate ➢ Use glasses/hearing aids as appropriate	➢ Side rails x 2 ➢ Low bed position ➢ Call light within reach ➢ Remove obstacles ➢ Glasses/hearing aids within reach as appropriate

☑ All of the required interventions for assessed risk above, have been completed

Foley present ☑

For high risk patients choose one or more of the following

- Video monitor ☑
- Room near nurse stat ☐
- Restraints ☐
- one to one ☐
- Pharmacy review ☑ Review Date: 3/2/2006

For moderate risk patients choose one or more of the following

- Gait belt ☐
- Up with assist ☑
- Bed Alarm ☐
- Pharmacy review ☑

Based on the shift assessment the following interventions are required: **Moderate Risk**

High Risk Interventions	Moderate Risk Interventions	Low Risk Intervention
➢ Red magnet on door jam ➢ Siderails x 4 ➢ Low bed position ➢ Bed alarm ➢ Every 30 minute checks ➢ Call light within reach ➢ Remove obstacles ➢ Encourage toileting q 1-2 hours (attended in bathroom at all times) ➢ Gait belt or up with assist when walking/standing ➢ Assess for use of Stedy device ➢ Adjust lighting as appropriate ➢ Use glasses/hearing aids as appropriate	➢ Side rails x 2 or 4 ➢ Low bed position ➢ Every hour checks ➢ Call light within reach ➢ Remove obstacles ➢ Offer toilet every 1-2 hours ➢ Assess for use of Stedy device ➢ Adjust lighting as appropriate ➢ Use glasses/hearing aids as appropriate	➢ Side rails x 2 ➢ Low bed position ➢ Call light within reach ➢ Remove obstacles ➢ Glasses/hearing aids within reach as appropriate

Other interventions selected in the shift assessment: Video monitoring; Pharmacy Review;

☑ All of the required interventions above remain in place

These screen shots offer a sample of what the fall-assessment screens look like at Poudre Valley Hospital.

Source: *Poudre Valley Hospital, Fort Collins, Colorado. Used with permission.*

safety trumps any personal discomfort—our first obligation is to keep our patients safe," Deflesen says.

"Some of our staff have an effective way of explaining why they must accompany the patient on what's generally seen as a private, personal activity," Deflesen explains. "One of our nurses makes a point of stressing to the patient that he will keep his head turned away and then takes the time during the bathroom session to explain the safety benefits of his being nearby by describing the falls that they are working diligently to avoid."

Video Monitoring

As an additional monitoring and reduction strategy, PVH began using video monitors on the neurosciences unit in February 2007. "We opted to add this extra measure for our population with the highest historical risk of falls," Deflesen explains.

Deflesen explains how the video monitoring works. "We have two nurses' stations on the unit, and we put the screens at the nurses' station that has more privacy. The video screens are monitored for no more than 3-hour sessions. When we see a patient start to come out of bed, we then page overhead on the unit the room number, and a staff member responds immediately." The success of the program is highly dependent on this immediate response. Staff are so used to this process now that when a room number is called out, they all know it is a fall-risk situation, and staff move immediately. Deflesen recommends that the video monitoring process use technology that lets you use low light, to see in the dark, and motion detection. He also recommends that staff not monitor more than 20 to 25 beds at any given time. Many falls happen at night, so being able to effectively monitor at night can make all the difference in this kind of monitoring system.

Seeing Improvements

"Our falls have come down a lot," Deflesen notes. He attributes this to the multifaceted falls-reduction approach used by PVH and to the culture of safety that is firmly supported at the hospital and by both leadership and staff. This engagement comes from a commitment to focusing on a systematic, standardized approach to patient safety from which PVH refuses to waver. "We're engaged in a major culture shift at the organization where our focus is on patient safety above all else," he notes. "It's not something you can opt out of," he continues. "You have to remain vigilant and focused on doing the right thing."

Deflesen says that another aspect of PVH's success in falls reduction has been in creating a transparent organization that shares its successes and challenges equally. "We have used storytelling as a way to share information and insight about falls-related experiences that have impacted our organization," he said. So far it seems to be working. PVH is seeing a reduction in falls, staff feel engaged and empowered to play their role to keep fall risk reduced, and the organization is seeing the benefits of embracing a culture of safety, resulting in improved outcomes for the patients they serve.

Strategy

Wireless fall monitor. Some organizations are having patients wear a small credit card–sized device on their thighs to alert nursing staff when a patient rises from bed. This can speed up response time for caregivers who may need to respond quickly to a high-risk patient. One organization found that its falls rate was reduced by 91% after using this device.[16]

Strategy

Bed alarms. In some instances, bed alarms are used to signal to nurses that a patient is standing up. These alarms are embedded in the mattress and a pad on the floor next to the patient's bed. These alarms can either signal by the bedside or can transmit wirelessly. In one case, an 18% reduction in falls was reported.

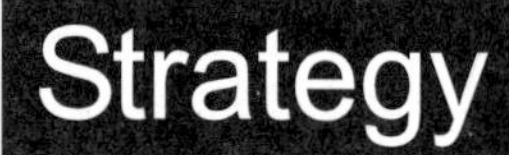

Passive fall-risk detection system. Some researchers are exploring ways to use sensors and passive monitoring systems to detect and alert when a patient has fallen. They are also looking at ways to monitor any changes in falls risk for a patient.

Strategy

Low-tech monitors. In some settings, affixing a "high-risk" identity to the patient can be helpful as a way to identify patients at risk for falls. Wearing a wristband may be preferable to posting signs in the patient's room, for example, in case the patient is moved. A wristband stays with the patient and can be easily identifiable.

Exercise and Nutrition

Some researchers are suggesting that a fall prevention program emphasizing exercise training or physical therapy may be more effective at preventing falls than more conventional approaches, such as education.[17] Researchers have also noted that although exercise may not improve older adult patients' anthropometrical and physical functioning, it did improve their falls self-efficacy. That same study suggested that the social activity of group exercise could also be attributed to improved outcomes for older adult patients.[17] Health care organizations can partner with local gyms or wellness centers to promote balance-building exercises, such as yoga and tai chi; long term care facilities may be able to provide such exercise for their ambulatory residents in their facilities.

Easing Patient Fears

The fear of falling (FOF) is a legitimate concern for older adult patients. Some patients will develop this fear after a fall, and others will develop a fear of falling without even having experienced a fall. The prevalence for fear of falling appears to increase with age and be predominant in women. Although FOF does exist in those who have previously fallen, having already experienced a fall was determined as a risk factor for developing the FOF. Less frequently mentioned were the risk factors of dizziness, depression, problems with gait and balance, low economic resources, and cognitive complaints.

FOF can result in significant changes in lifestyle. The negative impacts on FOF patients have been described as avoiding activities, experiencing depression, actually having falls, decreased social activity, and lower quality of life.[18]

Organizations, particularly in the ambulatory, home care, and long term care settings, can work with patients to assess their FOF risk and work with them to reduce the fear. If there is a physiological reason for the FOF, certain beneficial interventions could help: exercise, group activities, and physical therapy. In addition, because having had a previous fall is a known risk factor for FOF, implementing an effective fall-prevention program could go a long way toward easing a patient's FOF.

Educating Patients

Keeping patients safe from falls-related harm requires that they be educated and engaged in their own safety. Patients need to understand their own responsibility in keeping themselves safe and avoiding fall-risk hazards. The following important safety aspects should be stressed to patients:

- **Improve balance.** Encourage patients to pursue safe forms of exercise, such as tai chi, to help them improve balance and gain confidence in mobility.
- **Build strength.** Patients should understand that their strength can diminish with age. Muscle-building activities can be an important fall-prevention approach for patients.
- **Eat protein.** Another key element in building muscle comes from consuming healthy, low-fat amounts of protein. Patients can integrate protein into their diet.
- **Take Vitamin D.** Studies have linked taking Vitamin D with a reduction in falls.
- **Monitor medication and safety.** Encourage patients to understand and use medications wisely. Educate them on how to reconcile medication and how to ask their prescribing provider any questions if they are confused.
- **Check vision.** Because visual impairment has been linked to fall risk, patients should be encouraged to have their vision checked regularly.
- **Watch blood pressure.** Drops in blood pressure have been connected with an increase in falls. Patients should be encouraged to speak with their provider in the event that they have concerns over low blood pressure.
- **Check homes for safety.** With half of all falls taking place at home, patients should be encouraged and

educated on how to keep their home safe. Although an ambulatory health care organization may not be in a position to literally check a home for safety, if it determines one of its patients is at risk for falls due to a health condition or medication use, it can provide patient education and checklists for patients to work toward preventing falls. Consider sharing checklists like Table 2-1 on page 24 in Chapter 2.

Conclusion

A fall can occur quickly and, at times, unexpectedly, and it can have a dire outcome for the patient. But with solid assessment procedures and preventive techniques in place, a lot can be done to reduce the incidence of falls. Falls are a prevalent issue that need to be dealt with effectively to help reduce adverse affects for patients. The following chapter considers another area of safety concern for older adult patients: memory and mental health issues.

References

1. Medical News Today: http://www.medicalnewstoday.com/articles/126375.php (accessed Feb. 19, 2009).
2. Centers for Medicare and Medicaid Services: http://www.cms.hhs.gov/apps/media/press/release.asp?Counter=3041&intNumPerPage=10&checkDate=&checkKey=&srchType=1&numDays=3500&srchOpt=0&srchData=&srchOpt=0&srchData=&keywordType=All&chkNewsType=1%2C+2%2C+3%2C+4%2C+5&intPage=&showAll=&pYear=&year=&desc=&cboOrder=date (accessed Feb. 19, 2009).
3. National Center for Injury Prevention and Control. Division of Unintentional Injury Prevention: Falls among older adults: An overview. 2007. http://www.cdc.gov/ncipc/factsheets/adultsfalls.htm (accessed Mar. 22, 2009).
4. ECRI Institute: A snapshot of falls in healthcare settings: Falls prevention strategies in healthcare settings. Plymouth Meeting, PA: The Institute pp. 1–4, 2006.
5. Currie L.: *Fall and Injury Prevention in Patient Safety and Quality: An Evidence-Based Handbook for Nurses.* AHRQ Publication No. 08-0043. , Rockville, MD: Agency for Healthcare Research and Quality. http://www.ahrq.gov/qual/nurseshdbk/ (accessed Feb. 19, 2009).
6. Tiedemann A.C., et al.: Hospital and non-hospital costs for fall-related injury in community-dwelling older people. *NSW Public Health Bulletin* 19:9–10, 2008.
7. Leveille S.G., et al.: The MOBILIZE Boston study. *Geriatrics* 8:16, 2008.
8. Rubenstein L.Z., Josephson K.R.: Falls and their prevention in elderly people: What does the evidence show? *Med Clin North Am* 90:807–824, 2006.
9. Bulat T., et al.: Clinical practice algorithms: Medication management to reduce fall risk in the elderly—part 3, benzodiazepines, cardiovascular agents, and antidepressants. *J Am Acad Nurse Pract* 20:55–62, 2008.
10. Fisher K.: Floor maintenance: A scientific approach to slip/fall prevention. *Nursing Homes Magazine* pp. 80–82, Oct. 2007.
11. Hill K., et al.: Effectiveness of falls clinics: An evaluation of outcomes and client adherence to recommended interventions. *J Am Geriatr Soc* 56:600–608.
12. Shorr R.I., et al.: Improving the capture of fall events in hospitals. *J Am Geriatr Soc* 56:701–704, Apr. 2008.
13. Giles L.C., et al.: Can volunteer companions prevent falls among inpatients? A feasibility study using a pre-post comparative design. *Geriatrics* 6:11, 2006.
14. Fenton W.: Introducing a post-fall assessment algorithm into a community rehabilitation hospital for older adults. *Nurs Older People* 20(10):36–93, 2008.
15. Diduszyn J., et al.: Use of wireless nurse alert fall monitor to prevent inpatient falls. *J Clin Outcom Manag* 15:293–296, Jun. 2008.
16. Agnew T.: Downfall. *Nurs Older People* 20(1):6–7, 2008.
17. Fukukawa Y., et al.: Social support as a moderator in a fall prevention program for older adults. *J Geront Nurs* 34(5):19–25, 2008.
18. Scheffer A.C., et al.: Fear of falling: Measurement strategy, prevalence, risk factors and consequences among older persons. *Age Aging* 37:19–24, 2008.

Chapter 6

Memory, Mental Health Issues, and Older Adults

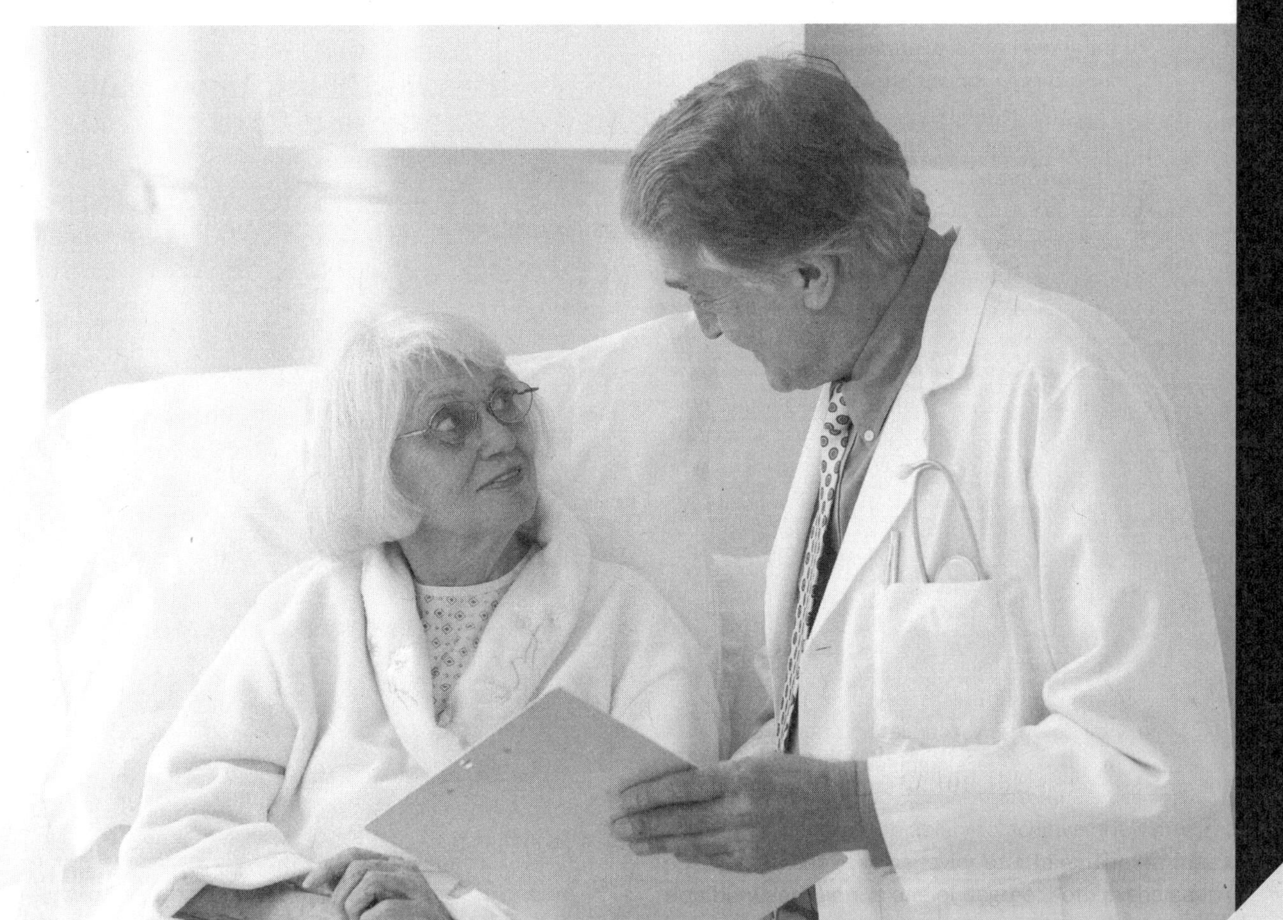

Memory and mental health issues have a significant impact on the quality of life and safety of older adult patients. Often, due to the symptoms and impact of such issues as dementia, depression, suicide ideation, and delirium, patients can face major safety risks.[1] To ensure that older adult patients remain safe, organizations should have processes in place to assess, monitor, and provide interventions to help reduce any chance of adverse outcomes for older adult patients, such as falls, adverse drug events (ADEs), wandering, infections, injury, and death.

Part of understanding memory and mental health issues is understanding the differences between what are often called the "3Ds": delirium, dementia, and depression. All these "Ds" impact patients in different ways. Depression, however, occurs at all ages, but it can manifest different symptoms and have a unique impact on an older adult patient. Understanding these symptoms can be particularly important to staff who are less experienced with caring for older adult patients. Consider the following table, Table 6-1, which outlines the signs and symptoms of delirium, depression, and dementia.

One important aspect of caring for older adult patients suffering from dementia or depression is assessment. Consider the following aspects of a detailed patient history:[1]

- Onset and duration of symptoms
- Recent stressful or traumatic events, such as surgery or a death in the family
- Head trauma
- Changes in the environment
- New medications, including over-the-counter products
- Dietary history
- Personal or family history of alcoholism or other substance abuse, dementia, depression, suicide or suicide attempts, or thyroid disease, which may be implicated in delirium (thyrotoxic crisis) or dementia (hypothyroidism)

These conditions can impact each other, such as in the case of delirium superimposed on dementia or depression complicating dementia. Consider the following in relation to how delirium and depression can complicate dementia:[1]

- Dementia plus delirium
  - If a dementia patient suddenly becomes agitated, he or she should be assessed for delirium. If delirium exists, assess for an underlying physical illness or disorder, such as infection, pain, fever, or constipation.
  - Because dementia patients may have trouble communicating, varied assessment strategies should be applied, such as patient observation, a physical exam, lab test results, patient history from family, surrogate decision makers, or medical records.
- Dementia plus depression
  - A patient in the early stages of dementia may be aware of cognitive changes and so may become depressed. Signs of depression include physical symptoms, feelings of hopelessness or suicidal ideation, abrupt mood changes, sleep disturbances, and changes in functional status.
  - With the progression of dementia, depression could become less noticeable.
  - If the use of antidepressants reduces symptoms, then a diagnosis of depression can be confirmed.

Understanding the relationship between these conditions and their impact on patient safety are important aspects of ensuring older adult patients remain as safe as possible.

Dementias and Their Impact on Patient Safety and Care

Dementia is not a normal expectation for an aging adult. It is a serious and progressive neurologic disorder impacting 10% of adults age 65 to 85, 20% of adults age 75 to 85, and 50% of adults over age 85. Alzheimer's disease represents 65% of dementia cases.[1]

Consider Sidebars 6-1 and 6-2 for strategies in communication with dementia sufferers (Sidebar 6-1) and for suggestions on nursing interventions for patients with dementia (Sidebar 6-2). In addition, Sidebar 6-3 includes a list of suggested interventions for specific behaviors that can happen with dementia patients.

Keeping Patients with Dementia Safe

Wandering Off

A facility-based patient with dementia poses a risk of wandering, for which organizations should plan. Any patient with dementia who is moving is said to be "wandering." This movement needs focus for the following reasons:

Table 6-1. Definitions, Symptoms, and Etiologies of Delirium, Dementia, and Depression

Disorder	Definition
Depression	A disorder that typically includes changes in feelings or mood, often described as feeling sad, hopeless, pessimistic, or "blue." A major depression is characterized by a depressed mood lasting at least 2 weeks and accompanied by clinically significant distress or impairment in social, occupational, or other important areas of function.
Delirium	Depressed level of conscious awareness, confused state. A disturbance of consciousness that is accompanied by a change in cognition that cannot be better accounted for by a pre-existing or evolving dementia.
Dementia	Diminished, irreversible changes in cognitive function, damage to the nervous system.

Clinical manifestation	
Depression	■ Dysphoria, changes in mood (for example, feeling sad, hopeless, pessimistic) ■ Loss of interest in life ■ Irritability and anxiety ■ Disorientation ■ Changes in appetite, weight ■ Changes in sleep/wake patterns ■ Changes in activity levels ■ Fatigue ■ Decreased motivation and interest in activities of daily living ■ Decreased libido ■ Decreased concentration and attention ■ Loss of short-term memory
Delirium	■ Sudden, short onset ■ Perceptual disturbance ■ Incoherent speech ■ Disturbed sleep/wake cycle ■ Changes in psychomotor activity ■ Disorientation ■ Decreased level of consciousness ■ Evidence of potential organic cause ■ Memory impairment (especially recent, immediate memory)

continued

Source: *Depression, Delirium, and Dementia in the Elderly Patient. http://findarticles.com/p/articles/mi_m0FSL/is_2_72/ai_64424336 (accessed Mar. 23, 2009).*

Table 6-1. Definitions, Symptoms, and Etiologies of Delirium, Dementia, and Depression (Continued)

Clinical manifestation (continued)	
Dementia	■ Slow progression, plateaus, no improvement ■ Loss of memory and cognition ■ Inability to pay attention or follow simple directions ■ Disorientation ■ Changes in motor ability ■ Impaired language ■ Physical deterioration ■ Sleep/wake disturbances ■ Altered pattern of behavior ■ Delusions and hallucinations ■ Changes in weight ■ No change in consciousness in early stages ■ Mood changes

Etiology	
Depression	■ Genetic predisposition ■ Female gender ■ Negative life events ■ Chemical imbalances ■ Therapeutic and recreational drugs ■ Postpartum changes ■ Previous episodes of depression ■ Older age
Delirium	■ Almost anything ■ Organic changes ■ Psychosocial changes ■ Environmental changes ■ Older age
Dementia	■ Alzheimer's disease ■ Multiple brain infarctions ■ Trauma ■ Drug, alcohol toxicity ■ Parkinson's disease ■ Nutritional deficiencies ■ Heavy metal poisoning ■ Pick's disease ■ Creutzfeldt-Jakob disease ■ Older age

Sidebar 6-1. Communication Strategies

Early and Middle Stages of Dementia

- Repeat messages frequently.
- Use short sentences.
- Ask one question at a time and allow plenty of time for a response.
- Break down instructions into separate components. "Put your arm in the sleeve." "Button up." "Tuck in your shirt tail."
- Provide written cues as reminders, because written messages are retained longer than spoken ones. For example, write out the person's schedule for the day rather than just telling him.
- Give directions close to the time the person must follow them (for example, within an hour rather than the morning or the day before).

Later Stages of Dementia

- Remind the person with dementia tactfully what he or she was talking about during a conversation.
- Make such things as familiar music, pictures, and scents available.
- Avoid asking open-ended questions, such as "What do you want to drink?" Rather, offer two choices whenever possible: "Do you want coffee or soda?"
- Remember that word recognition lasts longer than word recall; say aloud what you think the person is trying to say to see if the patient can signal whether you are correct.
- Use "fill-in-the-blanks" to help find the words. For example, if the person is trying to remember the word "butter," you might say "Pass the bread and ____."
- Avoid correcting wrong words.
- Allow the patient to write or spell words he cannot say.
- Avoid interrupting or rushing; allow time for processing and understanding.
- Look for clues to messages in facial expression, tone of voice, and behavior.
- Use a reassuring tone of voice with lots of touch and body language; the person may still understand a wave and an outstretched hand.
- Avoid saying things in the person's presence that you do not want the person to know; it is impossible to know how much she understands.
- Repeat the message frequently.
- Use simple words.
- Use short sentences; avoid using complex sentence structures.
- Allow time to finish one task before moving on to the next.
- Enhance your message with pictures, objects, gestures, and body language.
- Avoid competing messages, such as television, radio, other conversations; anticipate difficulties in large groups or with strangers.
- Speak slowly.
- Speak face-to-face, making eye contact.
- Use appropriate tone of voice for your message; avoid sending unintentional emotional signals by your manner of speaking.
- Use a calm, pleasant, inviting tone of voice; avoid addressing the person as a child.

Source: *Reprinted from* MEDSURG Nursing, *2004, Vol. 13, No. 1, pg. 23. Reprinted with permission of the publisher, Jannetti Publications, Inc., East Holly Avenue, Box 56, Pittman, NJ 08071-0056; Phone (856) 256-2300; Fax (856) 589-7463.*

- **Falls.** A disoriented or aimlessly wandering patient could be at a higher risk for falls.
- **Elopement.** Although not all wanderers will elope (unescorted exiting) from the facility, it can happen.

Consider the following suggestions for keeping a facility safe:[2]

Design of the building. Try to avoid letting dementia patients stay in areas where there are narrow, long hallways—dementia patients prefer open spaces where they can see where they are going. Place exits near the nursing stations so staff can intervene in the event of wandering.

Signage. Clear, easy-to-read signage can help patients reorient where they are going. Keep in mind such colors as red, yellow, or orange, which are easier for older adult patients to see.

Sidebar 6-2. General Nursing Interventions for Patients with Dementia

- Think about reasons that the behavior might be occurring. Is the patient hungry? Does she need to go to the bathroom? Is she in pain, worried?
- Tell the patient where he is, that he is safe, and that you are taking care of him.
- Try responding to the need behind the words. If the patient repeats, "I need to go home," over and over, this might suggest that she feels unsafe.
- Find out and share with others what has worked (or not worked) in the past, but be willing to try things that may not have worked before.
- Do things the same way, in the same order, every day.
- Encourage visits or telephone calls from friends and family.
- Distraction often helps to stop undesired behaviors. Try offering food or drink, watching television, listening to music, going for a walk or to an activity, or talking about something else (for example, things from the past). An audio or videotape of friends or family may also be a good distraction. Remember that many distractions can also be "noise" and actually cause problems.
- Physical touch may be helpful, or sometimes it can cause more problems. Use physical touch only if it is beneficial.

Source: *Reprinted from* MEDSURG Nursing, *2004, Vol. 13, No. 1, pg. 25. Reprinted with permission of the publisher, Jannetti Publications, Inc., East Holly Avenue, Box 56, Pittman, NJ 08071-0056; Phone (856) 256-2300; Fax (856) 589-7463.*

Alarms. Use door alarms that alert staff when an exit door is being opened or bed alarms that alert staff when a patient tries to get out of bed by him- or herself.

A "lost person" plan can be useful to develop in the event of an eloping patient. This is particularly useful in long term care facilities, where the incidence of dementia patients is more prevalent. The plan could include the following elements:[2]

- Accounting for patients on a regular basis
- A sign-in and sign-out process for patients' families and other visitors, especially when a patient leaves the facility
- Keeping a recent set of photos of patients on hand (particularly in a long term care setting)
- A process to inform authorities and families in the event of elopement
- An organized search plan
- A way to provide information on how to search for a patient with dementia
- Keeping information on hand for nearby bus terminals, train stations, or taxi services

Communicating Needs

Communicating with a dementia patient can be extremely difficult. It requires a flexible, adaptive "trial and error" approach to see what helps with communication. Although this can take extra time and effort on the part of care providers, striving to work with the patient on communicating his needs can go a long way toward ensuring his safety and care. Some techniques for communicating with dementia patients include:[3]

Look for emotions behind a patient's words. If she asks, "When is Mommy coming?" that may actually mean, "I'm frightened of this place and want to go home."

Use simple, concrete nouns and positive messages. "Your scarf is on the table" or "Stay sitting in the chair" are clear messages. Avoid ambiguous statements and slang.

Watch what you do. A dementia patient can pick up on body language and mood; use your voice and demeanor to send calming messages and remember to slow down to prevent agitation.

Sidebar 6-3. Interventions for Specific Behaviors

Wandering/Pacing:

- Offer to let the patient sit with staff at the nursing station. Use distraction. Encourage the patient to do a seated activity.
- Consider the physical layout of your unit or department and locate dementia patients near a corridor with a dead end so they can wander safely without the risk of elopement.
- Walk with the patient on walkways that are clear. Be alert for objects in the way or wet floors that might increase fall risk.

Repeated Actions

- Ignore the action if it is not harmful to the patient or others or not destructive of property.
- If behavior is harmful or destructive, or perhaps even if it is merely annoying to others, replace it with something else physical to do: folding towels, wiping tables, rolling yarn balls, tearing rags, or doing puzzles.

Resistance to Care

- First, approach the patient, then make eye contact. Next tell the patient what activity will be happening. Do not start care without first talking to the person.
- If possible, give care at a time of day good for the patient and when you do not have to hurry. If the patient is fighting care, postpone it, if possible, and try later.

Repeated Questions/Comments

- Do not discuss such things as visits or appointments until just before they will happen.
- Give simple answers to repetitious questions. Use memory aids, as appropriate: notes, signs, clocks, or calendars.

Screaming/Yelling

- Check to see if there are things that might be frightening or upsetting to the patient.
- First, be sure the person's needs are met (for example, she is not in pain, thirsty, hungry, or needing to go to the bathroom) and will be safe alone. Then inform the patient that you are going to give him or her a "time out" and specify the length of time (10 to 15 minutes). Next, promise to return and check on the patient at the end of that time. Also, promise to spend time with the patient if he or she does not scream or yell during the time out. Specify the length of time and what you'll do: talk, do an activity, and so on. Be sure to follow through on your promises, and, if possible, do not let anyone else go in during the time out.

Source: *Reprinted from* MEDSURG Nursing, *2004, Vol. 13, No. 1, pg. 26. Reprinted with permission of the publisher, Jannetti Publications, Inc., East Holly Avenue, Box 56, Pittman, NJ 08071-0056; Phone (856) 256-2300; Fax (856) 589-7463.*

Don't argue, scold, or quiz a patient. Stop if a topic is upsetting and try again later or use distraction to de-escalate any agitation.

Don't refer to actual "clock" time. Say "Lunch is here," rather than "It's twelve o'clock, lunch time!"

Home Safety for Dementia Patients

Keeping dementia patients safe in the home is an essential patient safety concern. In an unsafe environment, falls, ADEs, elopement, or injuries could take place. Consider the following tips on helping patients and their families ensure that their homes are safe for dementia patients:[4]

Remove sharp-edged furniture, keep electrical cords out of the way, ensure floors are safe and not slippery (remove throw rugs).

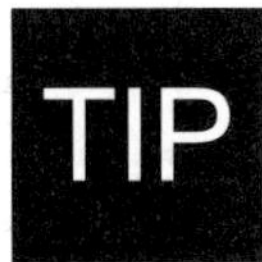

Use child-safety measures, such as childproof locks and doorknobs.

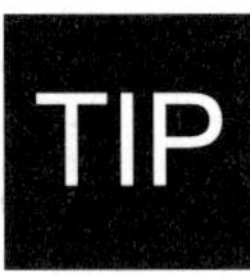

Store cleaning supplies, knives, and other potentially dangerous household goods in a safe, out-of-reach location.

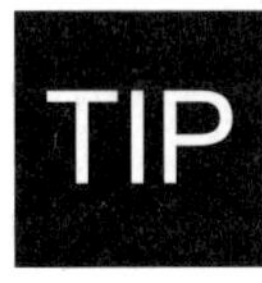

Keep all medications out of reach.

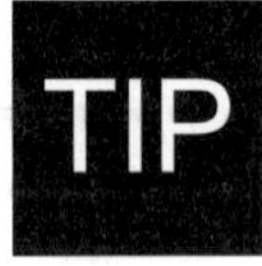

Use signage to help orient the patient.

Ensure the home contains working smoke alarms and a first-aid kit.

Surrogate Decision Makers

At the end of life or in the cases of cognitive impairment, patients may be incapable of making their own decisions about medical care. In these cases, surrogate decision makers may be asked to make significant decisions about a dementia patient, and this can be challenging for some individuals placed in this role. Studies have found that some surrogate decision makers experience post-traumatic stress due to difficult decisions made on behalf of their loved one.[5] Organizations should develop means to effectively work with surrogate decision makers to provide extensive information, help them understand their role, and help mitigate any negative impact on surrogate decision makers.

Depression and Its Impact on Older Adult Patient Safety and Care

Depression is not a older adult–specific disorder, but it can affect older adult patients. Some estimates say that up to one-third of older adult patients experience depression.[6] Consequences of depression include amplification of pain and disability, delayed recovery from illness and surgery, worsening of drug side effects, excess use of health services, cognitive impairment, subnutrition, and increased suicide- and nonsuicide-related death.[7] Organizations should have processes in place to help determine risk for depression and put in place interventions to help reduce risk.

Risk Factors for Depression

Risk factors for depression in older adult patients include:[6]

- Being female
- Widowed, divorced, or retired
- Over age 85
- Previous experience with depression
- Low socio-economic situation, poor housing, financial difficulties
- Low self-esteem
- A victim of crime or abuse
- Polypharmacy
- Use of alcohol or substances
- Pain
- Mobility problems
- Pressure ulcers, skin problems
- Loneliness and isolation
- Transition into long term care
- Early onset of dementia

Depression can have negative impacts on a patient's well-being and safety. It can cause the following:[8]

- Increased mortality
- Increased morbidity
- Excess functional disability
- Increased need for health care
- Increased somatic symptoms
- Poor self-care
- Decreased adherence to treatment and/or medicine
- Drug interaction dangers due to polypharmacy

Sidebar 6-4. Geriatric Depression Scale: Short Form

Choose the best answer for how you have felt during the past week. Answers in **bold** indicate depression. Score 1 point for each bolded answer.

1. Are you basically satisfied with your life? YES / **NO**
2. Have you dropped many of your activities and interests? **YES** / NO
3. Do you feel that your life is empty? **YES** / NO
4. Do you often get bored? **YES** / NO
5. Are you in good spirits most of the time? YES / **NO**
6. Are you afraid that something bad is going to happen to you? **YES** / NO
7. Do you feel happy most of the time? YES / **NO**
8. Do you often feel helpless? **YES** / NO
9. Do you prefer to stay at home, rather than going out and doing new things? **YES** / NO
10. Do you feel you have more problems with memory than most? **YES** / NO
11. Do you think it is wonderful to be alive now? YES / **NO**
12. Do you feel pretty worthless the way you are now? **YES** / NO
13. Do you feel full of energy? YES / **NO**
14. Do you feel that your situation is hopeless? **YES** / NO
15. Do you think that most people are better off than you are? **YES** / NO

A score > 5 points is suggestive of depression.
A score > 10 points is almost always indicative of depression.
A score > 5 points should warrant a follow-up comprehensive assessment.

Source: *Stanford University, Stanford, California, http://www.stanford.edu/~yesavage/GDS.html (accessed Feb. 24, 2009). Public domain.*

Intervening to Reduce the Risk of Depression

Researchers suggest that the following "protective factors" can make a difference in reducing the incidence of depression among older adult patients[6]:

- High degree of self-esteem
- High feelings and experience of mastery
- Presence of a confidant
- Positive social support that provides experiences of pleasure and mastery
- Life control
- Social responsibility, involvement, and reciprocity
- Engagement in social and community life
- Positive adjustment to poor health and self-management

An effective assessment for depression should look for the risk factors as mentioned above, along with any identified risk factors specific to your organization and previous experience with depression among older adult patients. One possible assessment tool is the Geriatric Depression Scale (*see* Sidebar 6-4, above).

Suicide Risk and Prevention

Suicide is a major concern in older adult patients. Research has found that older adult patients do not exhibit the same characteristics or attributes as younger adults with suicidal ideation.

The following have been identified as key suicide risks among older adult patients:[9]

- Recent stressful life events
- Presence of chronic or terminal illness with disability
- Recent bereavement or relationship breakdown
- Widow/widower
- Evidence of depression or loss of interest or loss of pleasure
- Evidence of withdrawal
- Warning of suicidal intent

- Evidence of a plan to commit suicide
- History of psychosis
- Evidence of persecutory voices/beliefs
- Family history of serious psychiatric problems or suicide
- Presence or influence of hopelessness
- Previous suicide attempt
- History of socioeconomic deprivation or financial worries
- History of alcohol and/or drug misuse

Because research has found that most older adult patients who commit suicide see their physicians within a few months of their death and more than one-third within the week of their suicide, an organization's reliable assessment of suicide risk and introduction of interventions may avert suicide.[10]

Suicide Prevention in Long Term Care Settings

Long term care settings are one of the places where suicide is a constant concern due to some of the health reasons for which older adults seek long term care. However, few studies have examined the correlation between suicide risk and residency in long term care. Most studies available on the topic were conducted before the advent of long term care alternatives in the 1990s, such as home care, and all reported on relatively few cases.[11]

One of the first studies reported a lower rate of suicide in nursing home residents age 70 and older than in community-dwelling elderly people. In contrast, another study reported a suicide rate in long term care residents age 60 and older substantially higher than in the general population.[11] The finding was replicated by a more recent study which found a higher rate of suicide in long term care residents age 65 and older than in the general regional population.[11]

There are also relatively few published studies on the methods used to complete suicide in long term care, which would be useful in prevention efforts. Suicide in older adults in the general U.S. population is frequently completed by using firearms, while the most commonly used method in long term care is hanging and jumping or falling.[11]

To better understand suicide among long term care residents, a study was done in New York over a 15-year period from 1990 to 2005. During this time, there were 47 suicides in residents of long term care facilities and 1,724 suicides in community-living adults age 60 and older in New York City.[11] The long term care group was relatively older than the community-dwelling group; however, in both groups, most decedents were male and non-Hispanic white. The distribution of methods used in long term care reflected the more restrictive nature of the setting. Suicides in long term care were less likely to be due to firearms and more likely to be due to a long fall than in community-dwelling older adults.[11]

The study concluded that it has been suggested that LTC facilities may protect persons from committing suicide because of the limited opportunities to perform the act because of high surveillance, less access to lethal means, greater burden of impairments that may impinge on the ability to execute a plan, and greater opportunity for health care providers to inquire about and intervene in the event of suicidal ideations. However, studies of predictors of nursing home admission suggest that older adults who reside in long term care have many of the characteristics associated with greater suicide risk and lower social support and depression. Dementia is the most prominent risk factor for admission to long term care, and cognitive impairment has been associated with suicide ideation. Also, anticipation of placement in long term care has been identified as a potential risk factor for suicide in older adults. Together, these findings suggest that placement in long term care may be an indicator of an accumulation of risk for suicide.[11]

The researchers suggest that future research should focus on identifying methods to reduce suicide risk in long term care residents. For example, suicide may be reduced by limiting resident access to high places, such as open windows and roofs, or using window guards. long term care residents should also be screened routinely and reassessed for psychiatric disorders that are associated with suicide risk, such as depression and dementia, and appropriately treated.[11]

Conclusion

With an ever-aging population, the "3Ds"—delirium, dementia, and depression—can have a negative impact on an older adult patient's well-being and safety. Because the signs and symptoms of the 3Ds are often overlapping, accurate assessments and understanding how to identify related risk factors are essential to prevent any adverse events that they may cause. In addition, such risks as suicide ideation can manifest in older adult patients differently from their younger counterparts, so organizations need to understand the differences and be able to effectively assess any risks. The following chapter discusses issues relating to elder abuse and neglect and what organizations can do to help assess for and prevent their incidence.

References

1. Arnold E.: Sorting out the 3D's: Delirium, dementia, depression. *Nursing* 34(6):36–42, 2004.
2. Tilly J., Reed P.: Caring for residents who wander. *Provider* pp. 61–69, Oct. 2006.
3. Hilgers J.: Comforting a confused patient. *Nursing* pp. 48–50, Jan. 2003.
4. When someone you love has Alzheimer's. 68(1):31, 2005. http://www.rnweb.com (accessed Feb. 24, 2009).
5. Vig E.K., et al.: Surviving surrogate decision-making: What helps and hampers the experience of making medical decisions for others. *J Gen Int Med* 22:1274–1279, 2007.
6. Waugh A.: Depression and older people. *Nurs Older People* 18(8):27–30, Sep. 2008.
7. http://consultgerirn.org/topics/depression/want_to_know_more (accessed Feb. 19, 2009).
8. Suter P., et al.: Depression revealed: The need for screening, treatment, and monitoring. *Home Healthcare Nurse* 26:543–550, Oct. 2008.
9. Garand L., et al.: Suicide in older adults: nursing assessment of suicide risk. *Issues Ment Health Nurs* 27:355–370, 2006.
10. Alexopoulos, G., et al.: Clinical determinants of suicidal ideation and behavior in geriatric depression. *Arch Gen Psychiatry* 56(11):1048–1053, 1999.
11. Mezuk B., et al.: Suicide in older adults in long term care: 1990 to 2005. *J Am Geriatr Soc* 56:2107–2111, 2008.

Chapter 7

Spotting Abuse or Neglect in Older Adults

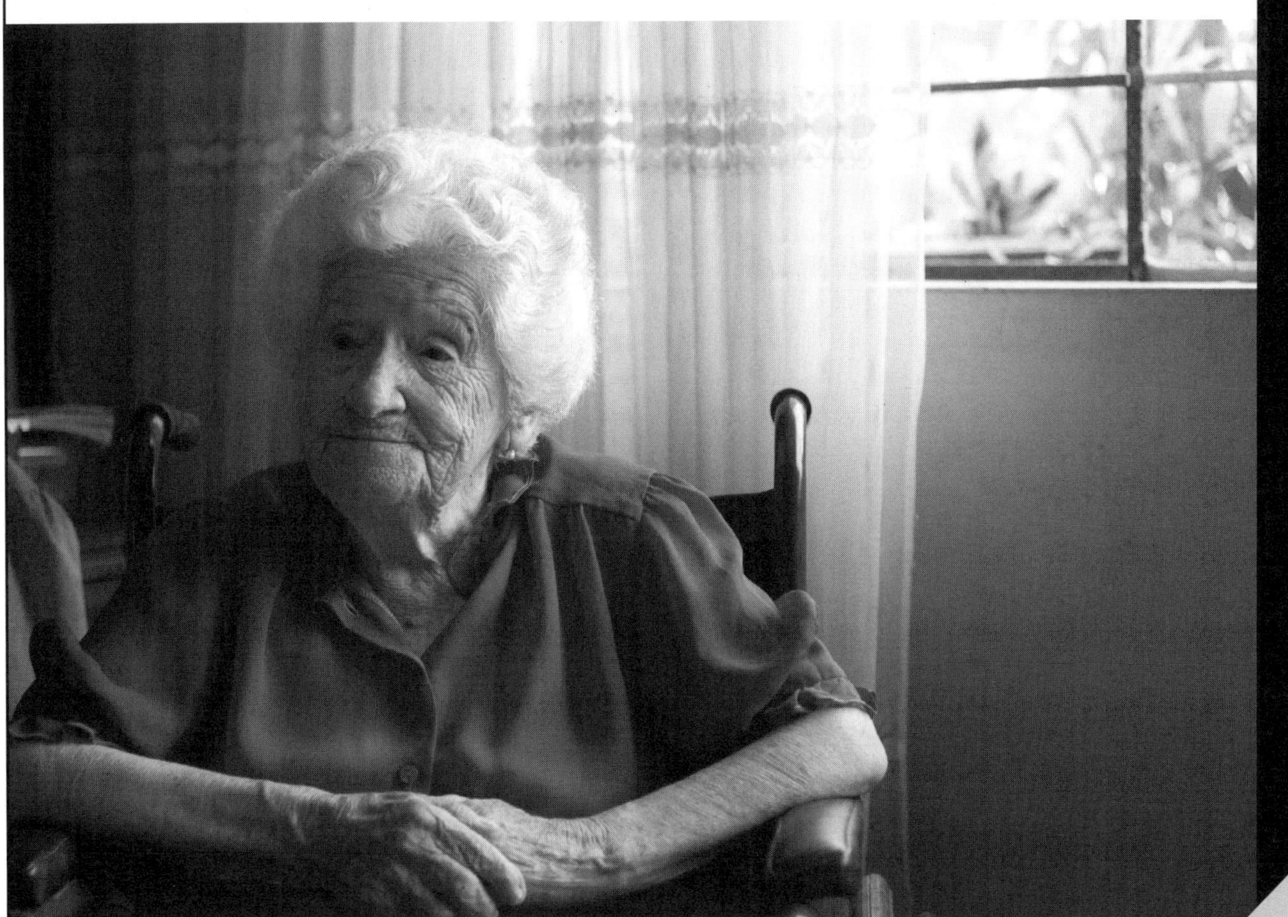

Abuse and neglect constitute a serious risk for geriatric patients. It is a serious problem that is often underreported and, in comparison to other vulnerable populations that may also be at risk for abuse and neglect, such as children and those with disabilities, appears underappreciated. Some estimates place the number of older Americans falling victim to abuse at 2.16 million a year.[1] And the challenge faced by health care organizations and authorities is that a lot of these cases go unreported. Although the actual incidence and prevalence of elder abuse in the United States are not known, one 1998 report estimated that for every case of elder abuse that is reported, another five go unreported.[1] The incidence of older adult patient abuse and neglect is not limited to the United States alone. One report estimated that at any given time in the general global population, almost 6.3% of elders are experiencing abuse.[2]

Neglect and self-neglect also pose significant threats to elders. In the case of an older adult patient with pre-existing health concerns and increased risk factors, the added threat of neglect or self-neglect genuinely challenges the safety of that patient.

Neglect and Abuse by Family Members

An interdisciplinary assessment and intervention plan for actual or potential elder abuse and neglect is essential to ensuring the safety and health of older adults in any clinical setting. Assessment and intervention should be directed toward both the victim and the alleged perpetrator. In many cases, an organization will need to abide by its state's regulations in relation to reporting cases of abuse, but prevention and assessment can be performed by an organization to help avoid abuse, if possible.

Risk factors for elder abuse include the following:

- Caregiver stress
- Childhood trauma
- Cultural sanctions against seeking help to care for elders
- Delirium
- Dependency of abuser on victim for housing and finances
- Dependence of elder on caretaker for assistance with activities
- Family history of violence
- Financial strain
- Increased age
- Isolation of the caregiver or victim
- Lack of close family ties
- Mental illness in family members/caretakers
- New, worsening, or prolonged depression
- New, worsening, or prolonged physical impairment
- Poverty/lack of financial resources
- Progressing dementia
- Shared living arrangement
- Substance abuse in family members/caretakers
- Unsafe living situation

The following physical findings are common in victims of abuse or neglect:

- Bruises
- Wounds
- Patterned injuries
- Poor nutrition
- Fractures
- Burns
- Genital lesions
- Anorectal findings
- Poor hygiene

Preventing abuse in older adult patients is of primary concern to organizations. Organizations can consider the following sidebar, Sidebar 7-1, page 93, for strategies to assess and intervene in cases of abuse.

Self-Neglect

In the case of self-neglect, an older adult patient will often have advanced undiagnosed and untreated medical and psychiatric conditions, including dementia and depression, in addition to living in squalor and having poor hygiene and nutritional status.[3]

The following represents the signs and symptoms of elder self-neglect:[4]

- Physical examination
  - Unkempt hair, nails, or clothes
  - Unexplained weight loss
  - Unusual wounds or odors
- Clinical signs
  - Missed medication refills or physician appointments
  - Decline in cognitive function
  - Frequent acute exacerbations of chronic illnesses and untreated medical diseases

Sidebar 7-1. Assessment and Intervention of Elder Abuse and Mistreatment

Type of Abuse/Mistreatment—Questions to Assess Type of Mistreatment Physical Assessment and Signs and Symptoms

Physical abuse:

- Has anyone ever tried to hurt you in any way?
- Have you had any recent injuries?
- Are you afraid of anyone?
- Has anyone ever touched you or tried to touch you without permission?
- Have you ever been tied down?

Suspected evidence of physical abuse (for example, a black eye):

- How did that get there?
- When did it occur?
- Did someone do this to you?
- Are there other areas on your body like this?
- Has this ever occurred before?

Assess for:

- ❑ Bruises (more commonly bilaterally to suggest grabbing)
- ❑ Black eyes
- ❑ Welts
- ❑ Lacerations
- ❑ Rope marks
- ❑ Fractures
- ❑ Untreated injuries
- ❑ Bleeding
- ❑ Broken eyeglasses
- ❑ Use of physical restraints
- ❑ Sudden change in behavior
- ❑ Note if a caregiver refuses an assessment of the older adult alone.
- ❑ Review any laboratory tests. Note any low or high serum prescribed drug levels.
- ❑ Note any reports of being physically mistreated in any way.

Emotional/Psychological abuse:

- Are you afraid of anyone?
- Has anyone ever yelled at you or threatened you?
- Has anyone been insulting you and using degrading language?
- Do you live in a household where there is stress and/or frustration?
- Does anyone care for you or provide regular assistance to you?
- Are you cared for by anyone who abuses drugs or alcohol?
- Are you cared for by anyone who was abused as a child? Assess cognition, mood, affect, behavior.

Assess for:

- ❑ Agitation
- ❑ Unusual behavior
- ❑ Level of responsiveness
- ❑ Willingness to communicate
- ❑ Delirium
- ❑ Dementia
- ❑ Depression
- ❑ Note any reports of being verbally or emotionally mistreated.

Sexual abuse:

- Are you afraid of anyone?
- Has anyone ever touched you or tried to touch you without permission?
- Have you ever been tied down?
- Has anyone ever made you do things you didn't want to do?
- Do you live in a household where there is stress and/or frustration?
- Does anyone care for you or provide regular assistance to you?

continued

Sidebar 7-1. Assessment and Intervention of Elder Abuse and Mistreatment (continued)

- Are you cared for by anyone who abuses drugs or alcohol?
- Are you cared for by anyone who was abused as a child?

Assess for:

- ❑ Bruises around breasts or genital area
- ❑ Sexually transmitted diseases
- ❑ Vaginal and/or anal bleeding or discharge
- ❑ Torn, stained, or bloody clothing/undergarments
- ❑ Note any reports of being sexually assaulted or raped.

Financial abuse/exploitation:

- Who pays your bills?
- Do you ever go to the bank with him or her?
- Does this person have access to your account(s)?
- Does this person have power of attorney?
- Have you ever signed documents you didn't understand?
- Are any of your family members exhibiting a great interest in your assets?
- Has anyone ever taken anything that was yours without asking?
- Has anyone ever talked with you before about this?

Assess for:

- ❑ Changes in money handling or banking practice
- ❑ Unexplained withdrawals or transfers from patient's bank accounts
- ❑ Unauthorized withdrawals using the patient's bank card
- ❑ Addition of names on bank accounts/cards
- ❑ Sudden changes to any financial document/will
- ❑ Unpaid bills
- ❑ Forging of the patient's signature
- ❑ Appearance of previously uninvolved family members
- ❑ Note any reports of financial exploitation.

Caregiver neglect:

- Are you alone a lot?
- Has anyone ever failed you when you needed help?
- Has anyone ever made you do things you didn't want to do?
- Do you live in a household where there is stress and/or frustration?
- Does anyone care for you or provide regular assistance to you?
- Are you cared for by anyone who abuses drugs or alcohol?
- Are you cared for by anyone who was abused as a child?

Assess for:

- ❑ Dehydration
- ❑ Malnutrition
- ❑ Untreated pressure ulcers
- ❑ Poor hygiene
- ❑ Inappropriate or inadequate clothing
- ❑ Unaddressed health problems
- ❑ Nonadherence to medication regimen
- ❑ Unsafe and/or unclean living conditions
- ❑ Animal/insect infestation
- ❑ Presence of lice and/or fecal/urine smell
- ❑ Soiled bedding
- ❑ Note any reports of feeling mistreated.

Self-neglect:

- How often to you bathe?
- Have you ever refused to take prescribed medications?
- Have you ever failed to provide yourself with adequate food, water, or clothing?

Assess for:

- ❑ Dehydration
- ❑ Malnutrition
- ❑ Poor personal hygiene
- ❑ Unsafe living conditions
- ❑ Animal/insect infestation
- ❑ Fecal/urine smell
- ❑ Inappropriate clothing
- ❑ Nonadherence to medication regimen

Table 7-1. Screening Questions to Assess Functional Domains of Capacity for Self-Care and Self-Protection

	Decisional Capacity		
Domains of Self-Care and Self-Protection	**Appreciation of Problems**	**Consequential Problem Solving**	**Executive Capacity (verification of task performance)**
Personal needs and hygiene: Bathing, dressing, toileting, and ambulation in home.	–Has it been difficult, or do you need assistance, to wash and dry your body or take a bath?	–If you had trouble getting into the bathtub, how could you continue to bathe regularly without falling?	–Physical examination of hair, skin, and nails. –Gait evaluation and screening for balance problems and recent falls.
Condition of home environment: Basic repairs/maintenance of living area and avoidance of safety risks.	–Do you have any trouble getting around your home due to clutter, furniture, or other items? –It is important to make basic repairs to one's home; do any parts of your home need repairs?	–What if your air conditioner [or heater] stopped working; how would you fix the problem?	–Proxy reports of the home environment or a home safety evaluation performed by an occupational therapist or home health service.
Activities for independent living: Shopping and meal preparation, laundry and cleaning, using telephone and transportation.	–Going to the store is important for buying food and clothing for everyday life. Do you have any problems going to the store regularly?	–If you need to call a friend [a cab or other service] to take you to the store, how would you do that?	–Ask patient to use the clinic's phone and call a friend or other service to ask for a ride. [Patient should demonstrate all steps for making a call and getting information.]
Medical self-care: Medication adherence, wound care, and appropriate self-monitoring.	–People who forget to take their medications may end up having a worse health condition or need to see the doctor more often. Do you have problems remembering to take medications?	–Consider if you had to have someone give your medications to you and watch you take them. How would this affect your everyday life?	–Ask patient to bring all medication bottles from home, even empty ones. Review medication fill and refill dates and pill counts, or have a home-health nurse do a home medication assessment.
Financial affairs and estate: Managing checkbook, paying monthly bills, and entering binding contracts.	–What difficulties do you have paying your monthly bills on time? –Who can assist you with paying your monthly bills or managing your finances?	–How could asking [cite individual] to help you with paying your bills be better than managing your monthly income and paying bills by yourself? –Are there any reasons why asking [cite individual] to manage your income might not help or might make things worse for you?	–Proxy reports of bank statements, uncollected debts, or bills. Can formally assess performance with routine financial tasks, such as one- or three-item transactions, including making change or conducting a payment simulation using a check and register.

- Proxy reports
  - Dangerous or unkempt home
  - Unpaid bills and debts or evidence of exploitation
  - Functional decline in activities of daily living

Table 7-1 on page 95 includes screening questions to help determine function in an older adult patient suspected of self-neglect.

In many cases, severe cases of self-neglect may require intervention from social services or another agency and focused clinical care. One way to prevent self-neglect is to work with the older adult patient on any underlying conditions, such as depression, that may be triggering the self-neglect. Organizations can also ensure that the patients they serve have good nutritional status; are being supported socially by family, friends, and other affiliations (such as religious institutions); and are in a safe environment. Because other situations, such as being debilitated from a fall or pressure ulcer, can trigger depression and self-neglect in older adult patients, the overriding goal of promoting patient safety through a reduction in adverse events is likely to help reduce the incidence of self-neglect.

Resident-to-Resident Aggression in Long Term Care Settings

Resident-to-resident aggression (RRA) between long term care residents includes negative, aggressive physical, sexual, or verbal interactions that in a community setting would likely be construed as unwelcome. These interactions have high potential to cause physical or psychological distress as well as serious consequences for aggressors and victims.

RRAs can be a serious and difficult issue to face as a caregiver in a nursing home. Aggressive behaviors can be verbal (yelling, cursing, name calling) or physical (hitting, pushing). These events can occur without any provocation or because of a misinterpretation of facts or situations. Caregivers must be able to respond appropriately when one resident begins arguing or fighting with another resident.

Take, for example, residents living in an Alzheimer's care center. These residents are confused due to the cognition loss that they are experiencing from the disease process. A roommate, for example, is a stranger that he or she has likely never met before. He or she is now sharing this space with someone whom he or she is expected to trust automatically. If the resident is already experiencing paranoia, then becoming accustomed to sharing his or her space may even be more of a challenge. When this is tied together with the fact that all the residents are living with the same cognition loss and confusion about living in an unfamiliar place, the situation may be fertile for aggression.

Caregivers must approach the situation in a calm manner. Typically residents with dementia suffer from lability. They will mirror the emotions of those around them. If caregivers rush into a situation yelling, pushing, or threatening, the resident will become even more aggressive. Caregivers must try to identify the immediate cause of the agitation. Caregivers should focus on feelings and not facts. Validate what the person is feeling and help put those feelings into words. After a caregiver has been able to put those feelings into words, then use redirection to help refocus the energy onto a new task.

The best way to eliminate RRAs is prevent them before they occur. Programming is the key to success with this goal. Caregivers should integrate as much of a resident's past interests into his or her current daily schedule as possible. This will not only help the resident feel as though he or she has a purpose, it will also prevent boredom. The need for a purpose does not diminish as a person's dementia progresses. In fact, staying focused with purpose is as important in the late stages of the disease process as in the early stage.

Caregivers need to remember the following important tips in dealing with RRAs:[5]

- Never raise your voice to the residents fighting.
- Focus on the feelings, not on the facts.
- Limit distractions during the incident.
- Validate feelings and help put those feelings into words.
- Shift focus onto another activity.

Reporting

Organizations should have processes in place to report on older adult patient abuse. Consider the resource list in the Appendix, pages 114–115, for a list of agencies that handle abuse reports.

Conclusion

Elder abuse can take on many forms—physical, emotional, verbal, sexual, or financial—and can have a detrimental effect on the health and well-being of an older adult patient. And often a health care organization or health care provider can have a unique role to play in detecting abuse and helping put in steps to mitigate its impact. In addition, older adult patients can often face the daunting risk of abandonment and neglect and can even be the cause of their own self-neglect. Staff should to be well trained to use effective assessment to spot the signs of these potentially devastating cases and can often make the difference in breaking the cycle of abuse, neglect, or self-neglect. Chapter 8 continues to explore issues of older adult patient safety by considering special areas of concern to this vulnerable population: pressure ulcers, wound care, and incontinence.

References

1. Plitnick K.R.: Elder abuse. *AORN J* 87: 422–427, Feb 2008.
2. Naik A.D., et al.: Assessing capacity in suspected cases of self-neglect. *Geriatrics* 63(2):9–12, Feb. 2008.
3. Cooper C., Selwood A., Livingston G.: The prevalence of elder abuse and neglect: A systematic review. *Age Ageing* 37:151–160. http://ageing.oxfordjournals.org/cgi/content/full/37/2/151 (accessed Mar. 22, 2009).
4. Dyer C.B., Goins A.M.: The role of interdisciplinary geriatric assessment in addressed self-neglect of the elderly. *Generations* 24(2):23–27, 2000.
5. Alzheimer's Care Group: http://alzcaregroup.wordpress.com/2008/08/08/resident-to-resident-altercations/ (accessed Feb. 19, 2009).

Chapter 8

Special Needs and Older Adults

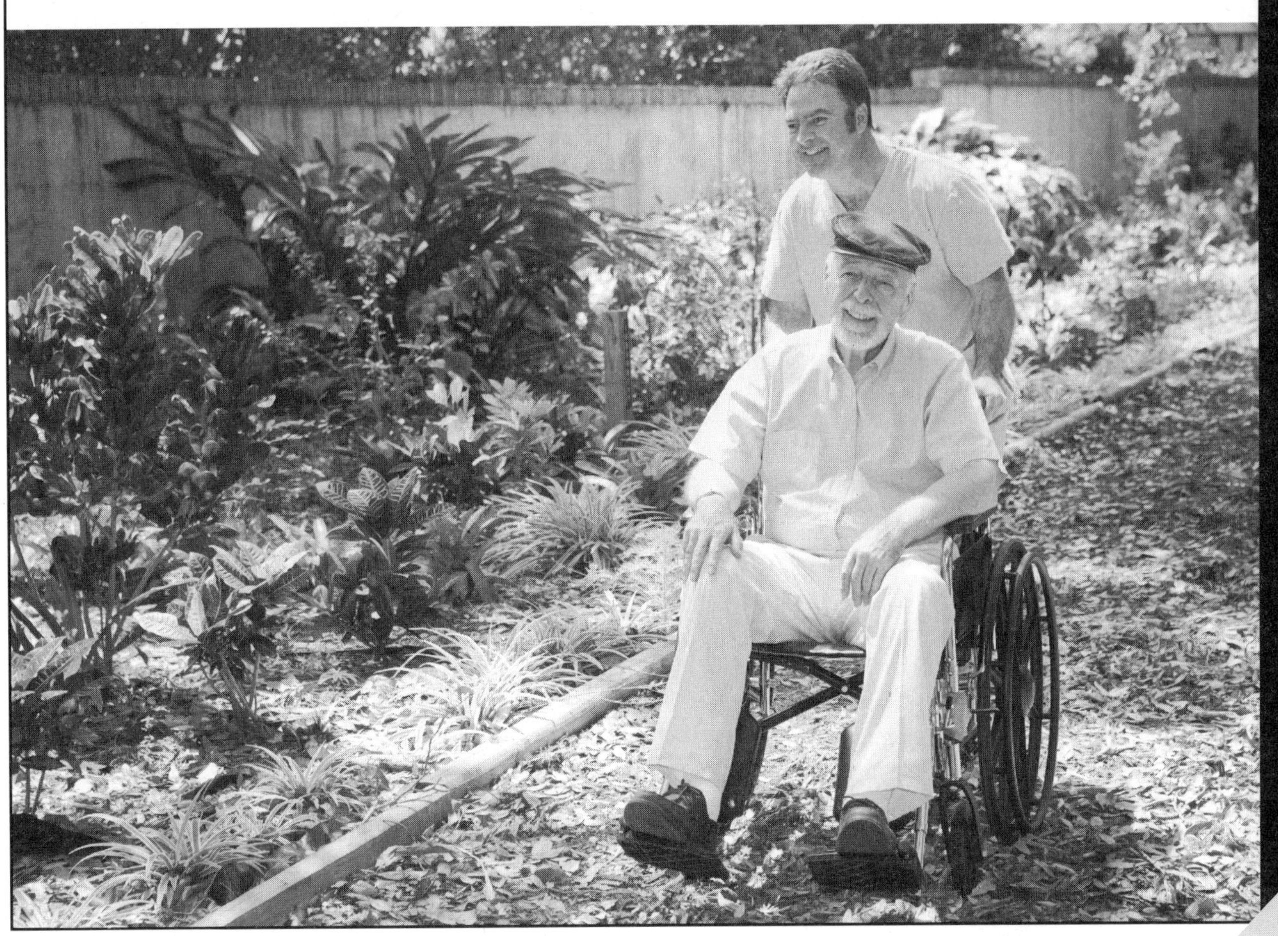

As this book has identified throughout, older adult patients face special needs and concerns regarding their health care and safety. Concerns relating to pressure ulcers and skin care, wound care, incontinence, poor nutrition, and dehydration require special consideration in relation to older adult patients, because they can either hasten other problems or contribute to functional decline in patients. It is not that these needs and concerns are unique to older adult patients, however, only that they and their potentially adverse outcomes can impact older adult patients on a more frequent basis, causing them added concern over their safety. The following risk factors can play into an older adult patient developing health care problems that could impact his or her well-being and safety:

- Advanced age
- Acute and chronic disease and illness
- Functional limitations
- Cognitive impairment
- Decreased (or lack of) mobility
- Frailty
- Deconditioning

This chapter concentrates on some special needs that older adult patients face and provides some tips and strategies on ways to deal with them in your organization.

Pressure Ulcers: Prevention and Care

Pressure ulcers are not a new phenomenon in health care; in fact, preventing pressure ulcers has long been a concern for nursing care. But despite this, their incidence is alarmingly on the rise in health care organizations. In 2004, there were pressure ulcers noted in 455,000 hospital stays, as compared to their appearance in 280,000 hospital stays in 1993. Between 1993 and 2003, the Healthcare Cost and Utilization Project report noted a 63% rise in pressure ulcers, while the total number of hospitalizations in that same time period rose by only 11%. This means that pressure ulcers are more common now than ever, and their incidence is often described as a failure in the entire health care team. For the older adult patient suffering with a pressure ulcer, the experience causes pain, limits activity, increases the risk of sepsis, and can degrade self-image.[1] Research indicates that among those patients experiencing pressure ulcers, there is a reported incidence from 0.4% to 38% in acute care, from 0% to 17% in home care, and from 2.2% to 23.9% in long term care.[2] The International Pressure Ulcer Prevalence Survey estimates that the prevalence of pressure ulcers in acute care is approximately 13.9%, although results have been found to vary significantly between countries, such as in the case of the Netherlands and Germany, where the prevalence of pressure ulcers was six times higher in the Netherlands as compared to Germany.[3,4]

The cost of treating a pressure ulcer is high: Recent estimates report an average cost of $37,800 per average hospital stay. In addition, some studies have noted a connection between pressure ulcers and mortality. Although a pressure ulcer was often not the cause of death, its existence signaled a decline in health status for an older adult patient and in some cases up to a 60% mortality rate has been reported.[5] Effective October 1, 2008, the Center for Medicaid and Medicare Services has stopped reimbursing hospitals for hospital-acquired conditions, which includes hospital-acquired Stage III and IV pressure ulcers.

Although preventing pressure ulcers is often a function of nursing care, research has suggested that when health care workers function as a team, the incidence of pressure ulcers has been decreased.[5] That team has to function effectively and rapidly. Not only are most pressure ulcers found to develop within the earlier parts of a patient's experience in a health care organization, but pressure ulcers themselves can develop within 2 to 6 hours. Thus, the assessment and identification of older adult patients who are at risk for developing pressure ulcers must be done early and effectively.

Although numerous risk factors have been identified for pressure ulcers, the American Medical Directors Association (AMDA) notes the following risk factors in particular for developing pressure ulcers:[6]

- Comorbid conditions, such as diabetes mellitus, end-stage renal disease, or thyroid disease
- Drugs that may affect ulcer healing, such as steroids
- Exposure of the skin to urinary or fecal incontinence
- History of a healed Stage III or IV pressure ulcer
- Impaired diffuse or localized blood flow, such as generalized atherosclerosis or lower-extremity arterial insufficiency
- Impaired or decreased mobility and functional ability
- Increase in friction or shear
- Moderate to severe cognitive impairment
- Patient refusal of some aspects of care or treatment
- Undernutrition, malnutrition, and hydration deficits

Figure 8-1. Braden Scale for Predicting Pressure Sore Risk

BRADEN SCALE FOR PREDICTING PRESSURE SORE RISK

Patient's Name ______________ Evaluator's Name______________ Date of Assessment

SENSORY PERCEPTION ability to respond meaning-fully to pressure-related discomfort	**1. Completely Limited** Unresponsive (does not moan, flinch, or grasp) to painful stimuli, due to diminished level of con-sciousness or sedation. OR limited ability to feel pain over most of body	**2. Very Limited** Responds only to painful stimuli. Cannot communicate discomfort except by moaning or restlessness OR has a sensory impairment which limits the ability to feel pain or discomfort over ½ of body.	**3. Slightly Limited** Responds to verbal com-mands, but cannot always communicate discomfort or the need to be turned. OR has some sensory impairment which limits ability to feel pain or discomfort in 1 or 2 extremities.	**4. No Impairment** Responds to verbal commands. Has no sensory deficit which would limit ability to feel or voice pain or discomfort..				
MOISTURE degree to which skin is exposed to moisture	**1. Constantly Moist** Skin is kept moist almost constantly by perspiration, urine, etc. Dampness is detected every time patient is moved or turned.	**2. Very Moist** Skin is often, but not always moist. Linen must be changed at least once a shift.	**3. Occasionally Moist:** Skin is occasionally moist, requiring an extra linen change approximately once a day.	**4. Rarely Moist** Skin is usually dry, linen only requires changing at routine intervals.				
ACTIVITY degree of physical activity	**1. Bedfast** Confined to bed.	**2. Chairfast** Ability to walk severely limited or non-existent. Cannot bear own weight and/or must be assisted into chair or wheelchair.	**3. Walks Occasionally** Walks occasionally during day, but for very short distances, with or without assistance. Spends majority of each shift in bed or chair	**4. Walks Frequently** Walks outside room at least twice a day and inside room at least once every two hours during waking hours				
MOBILITY ability to change and control body position	**1. Completely Immobile** Does not make even slight changes in body or extremity position without assistance	**2. Very Limited** Makes occasional slight changes in body or extremity position but unable to make frequent or significant changes independently.	**3. Slightly Limited** Makes frequent though slight changes in body or extremity position independently.	**4. No Limitation** Makes major and frequent changes in position without assistance.				
NUTRITION usual food intake pattern	**1. Very Poor** Never eats a complete meal. Rarely eats more than ⅓ of any food offered. Eats 2 servings or less of protein (meat or dairy products) per day. Takes fluids poorly. Does not take a liquid dietary supplement OR is NPO and/or maintained on clear liquids or IV's for more than 5 days.	**2. Probably Inadequate** Rarely eats a complete meal and generally eats only about ½ of any food offered. Protein intake includes only 3 servings of meat or dairy products per day. Occasionally will take a dietary supplement. OR receives less than optimum amount of liquid diet or tube feeding	**3. Adequate** Eats over half of most meals. Eats a total of 4 servings of protein (meat, dairy products per day. Occasionally will refuse a meal, but will usually take a supplement when offered OR is on a tube feeding or TPN regimen which probably meets most of nutritional needs	**4. Excellent** Eats most of every meal. Never refuses a meal. Usually eats a total of 4 or more servings of meat and dairy products. Occasionally eats between meals. Does not require supplementation.				
FRICTION & SHEAR	**1. Problem** Requires moderate to maximum assistance in moving. Complete lifting without sliding against sheets is impossible. Frequently slides down in bed or chair, requiring frequent repositioning with maximum assistance. Spasticity, contractures or agitation leads to almost constant friction	**2. Potential Problem** Moves feebly or requires minimum assistance. During a move skin probably slides to some extent against sheets, chair, restraints or other devices. Maintains relatively good position in chair or bed most of the time but occasionally slides down.	**3. No Apparent Problem** Moves in bed and in chair independently and has sufficient muscle strength to lift up completely during move. Maintains good position in bed or chair.					
				Total Score				

Source: *Copyright Barbara Braden and Nancy Bergstrom, 1988. Reprinted with permission.*

A number of risk assessment tools have been developed to help organizations determine risk for pressure ulcers. One example is the Braden Scale for Predicting Pressure Sore Risk, which is widely used. Figure 8-1 includes the tool.

Pressure ulcers can be prevented by applying a consistent approach. Consider the following recommended pressure ulcer prevention measures from the AMDA's *Pressure Ulcer Clinical Practice Guidelines*:[6]

- Create a turning and positioning schedule that is based on the patient's individual risk factors.
- Do not massage reddened areas over bony prominences.
- Evaluate and manage urinary and fecal incontinence.
- Initiate a plan to prevent or manage a contracture.
- Inspect skin during bathing or daily personal care.
- Maintain adequate nutrition and hydration if possible.
- Maintain the lowest possible head elevation to reduce the impact of shear.
- Position the patient to minimize pressure over bony prominences and shearing forces over the heels and elbows, base of head, and ears.
- Use appropriate offloading or pressure-redistribution devices.
- Use lifting devices, such as draw sheets or trapeze.
- Use proper transferring techniques.

Preventing pressure ulcers requires a focused, team-based approach. Consider the following tips to implement an effective pressure ulcer prevention strategy:[7]

Leadership and staff buy-in and support. Research has found that those organizations that have seen good success in reducing pressure ulcers have benefited from buy-in by both leadership and staff.

Organization champions. Any long-term effort, particularly one such as reducing pressure ulcers, can require a focused, organizationwide commitment. Having champions from different departments and from all disciplines can help reinforce the importance of the initiative and ensure that staff are engaged in it.

Keep things straightforward and consistent. Whatever your organization decides to do to prevent ulcers, ensure that the process is straightforward for staff to follow. Overly complicated documentation or assessment could put staff in the position where they create workarounds to the process.

Keep the solutions organization specific. Organizations have many resources to go to for information on preventing pressure ulcers, but the best approach for careful assessment of what works best in the organization, and for the individuals served, is related specifically to that organization.

Focus on the skin. Skin assessment and wound care is crucial to ensure patients stay healthy and avoid developing pressure ulcers. Skin assessment should be thorough.

Introduce multiple interventions. Some studies note that introducing a number of interventions can be helpful in reducing pressure ulcers, including the following examples:

- Total body system assessment
- Use of an electronic medical record with risk assessments built in
- Use of equipment for pressure relief
- Varied repositioning techniques (with staff training)
- Interdisciplinary team work
- Staff trained to be wound care specialists

Wound Care

Linked with the reduction of pressure ulcers is effective wound care. Wounds are not an unusual occurrence for a health care organization, but if left untreated or improperly

CASE STUDY

Spotlight on Improvement: Pocono Medical Center's Wound Care and Pressure Ulcer Prevention

When PMC, located in East Stroudsburg, Pennsylvania, learned that some of its patients were entering the hospital with wounds not being addressed in a timely manner, the hospital began a focused effort to improve on this potential patient safety problem. "Our investigation revealed that our skin assessment process in the emergency department (ED) was not being done consistently," explains Lisa Day, R.N., director nursing quality/education and research at PMC. Pocono's ED is extremely busy, so improving on the skin assessment and wound care process was essential.

Identifying Improvements

This knowledge came about when PMC conducted a failure modes and effects analysis (FMEA) in early 2008 on pressure ulcers. "Not only did the process work well, but it taught us that we had some issues with pressure ulcers that were linked to skin assessment and communication," notes Day. PMC wasted no time and began to make improvements.

Catherine Koch, R.N., certified wound ostomy and continence nurse and ostomy services manager for PMC, was responsible for improving the skin assessment and wound care process in the ED. The first step to implement was using an evidence-based skin assessment approach, particularly to assess the risk for pressure ulcers. "We use the reverse Braden assessment tool," Koch explains. "The higher the score, the higher the risk." (*See* the Braden tool on page 101.)

After PMC determines that the patient has a high risk for a pressure ulcer, the ED immediately responds by placing the patient on an air mattress and affixes a white armband on the patient that says "skin risk." "[His or her chart is then] flagged with a bright pink card to let the nurses know they have to perform wound measurements and staging," explains Koch. This helps the transition from assessment in the ED to transfer to a unit and is a helpful means of effective communication.

Designing Change

In addition, PMC uses a wound care flow sheet (*see* Figure 8-2 on page 106) and an interdisciplinary plan of care (*see* Figure 8-3 on page 107) for the wound care. The plan of care was designed by an interdisciplinary team. "We've had input from the unit clerks, technicians, physical therapy, nurses, case managers, physician assistants, and doctors on what the plan of care should include," notes Koch.

When it came to designing the flow sheet and plan of care, Koch notes a few important lessons learned from the planning process. "Know your population," she stresses. "Make sure that whatever you design is appropriate to whomever you serve." She also suggests that whatever assessment form you use, it should be as straightforward and easy to use as possible.

Above all, whatever plan or process is put in place, Koch stresses the importance of having direct care staff involved as a member of the team. "We found that active engagement with direct care staff helped a lot, because we had their buy-in to the process," she says.

Another thing Koch noticed was that some nurses needed additional training on skin assessment and wound care. "We spent time working with staff to ensure that they were able to effectively assess and stage wounds," Koch notes. "We wanted to be sure the staff knew the difference between diaper rash versus a Stage I pressure ulcer, for

At-a-Glance

About the hospital: PMC, located in East Stroudsburg, Pennsylvania, is a midsized, community hospital that serves a diverse population, including its older adult population.

About the improvement: When PMC noticed that some of its patients were entering the hospital without wounds being addressed in a timely manner, the medical center began a focused effort to improve its wound assessment and care process through education, training, and staff empowerment activity.

example." This was greatly aided by Koch's own specialized skill background in ostomy. Koch notes that the following areas were focused on in additional staff training:

- *Pressure ulcer prevention.* "There are some great educational resources online, such as the NPUAP Web site [http://www.npuap.org]," Koch notes. Koch points to the fact that NPUAP include visual aids for educational purposes.
- *Regular staff communication.* "We provide ongoing education for staff by sharing a 'wound care fact of the month,'" Koch notes. PMC also has posted alerts on each floor and has printed full-sized and pocket-sized guides on pressure ulcer nursing care guidelines and staging (*see* Figure 8-4 on page 108). Koch also stresses the importance of being able to document when a wound was healed. "Focusing on the positive means a lot to our staff and goes a long way toward continued diligence," she says.
- *Documentation.* PMC also has a "Skin Management Turning Schedule" sheet to track patient turns. PMC has designed a pad of paper with the body on it so the technicians and nurses' aides can note any changes in skin condition (*see* Figure 8-5 on page 109).

Leadership Support

Day points to the importance of this project to PMC and leadership's buy-in from the start. "The support has been strong at all levels," she explains. "We've even made a point to discuss the team and its achievements in the board meeting." Day notes that the board has been extremely involved in the hospital's quality improvement efforts.

A crucial aspect of the success of this work has been engaging the ED staff in the improvement efforts. "The ED staff did a great job of helping us identify what was realistic and manageable for them to effectively do the assessment," says Koch. "They were supportive and actually became engaged sooner than I would have originally anticipated."

But not every detail has worked as originally planned. Koch stresses the importance of knowing the culture of your organization and limits when implementing a change: "We had initially developed a physician order set for wound care and staging, but it proved too confusing and ineffective, so we stopped using it." Being flexible and making suitable changes is important to any effort like this, Koch points out.

The Next Step: Discharge

The next goal for PMC is working on its discharge process, particularly in relation to proper patient education on wound care and in communication with the outside agencies that the patient may be discharged to such as to home care or long term care.

An important aspect of this discharge improvement plan is engaging the communitywide health care organizations in the improvement planning. "We are now including our community home care agencies and long term care facilities in our skin care team," notes Koch. The first stage is when PMC hosts a diabetic wound care fair where all the local area organizations have been invited to participate. After that, PMC's skin care team will host its first team meeting with the communitywide representatives also involved.

Tracking Progress

The entire process began in January 2008 when PMC conducted its FMEA. By August 2008, PMC had its new assessment and wound care plan firmly in place. Six months into the new process, Day could already report improvements. "Our hospital-acquired prevalence of pressure ulcers has been only 1%," notes Day. "This is a dramatic improvement from where we were before at 4% to 7%." Day is encouraged by the initial findings but notes that the goal is zero.

Day notes that another goal for PMC is patient and family involvement in preventing pressure ulcers. "We have a patient/family communication option that we call 'code H,'" she says. "This allows families to call for help if they don't feel their family member's needs are being met." So far, the concerns raised by families in this process have been pain management related, but Day notes that the "code H" system may allow for more patient and family involvement in skin care.

Lessons Learned

Koch and Day offer the following suggestions to organizations looking to improve their own pressure ulcer prevention and skin assessment efforts.

Find an effective way to communicate wound care instructions on discharge. Koch and Day stress the value of having a streamlined, easy-to-read set of instructions for patients, particularly those who may be discharged from the hospital but not into home care.

Be open to doing things differently. Do not be too worried about how staff will adapt to a new process—they can often get excited if they feel engaged and brought into the process.

Make sure things are specific to your culture and organization.

The frontline staff are your champions and the best voice of support for a new process to other staff.

With a firm process already in place, and a plan to engage all communitywide organizations into their skin assessment and wound care processes, PMC and Monroe County, Pennsylvania, appear well positioned to dramatically reduce the risk of pressure ulcers among their patients.

cared for, they can develop into more serious conditions, such as pressure ulcers. Effective wound care, then, becomes a crucial patient safety endeavor that organizations should link to their pressure ulcer prevention efforts.

In the case of some organizations, the training of staff specialized in wound care or using a multidisciplinary wound care team has proven helpful. There are a number of effective approaches for treating chronic wounds:[8]

- Moist wound dressings, when appropriate, to assist healing
- Holistic approaches to local and systemic factors that prevent healing
- Specialized training in wound and skin care
- Having a wound care multidisciplinary team in place

Consider these additional suggestions for effective wound care:[9]

- Keep the skin clean and dry, and use skin protecting products. Reinforce good nursing practice in wound care.
- Conduct skin assessments. The Centers for Medicare & Medicaid Services (CMS) recommends that the following five elements be included:
    1. Skin temperature
    2. Color
    3. Turgor
    4. Moisture status
    5. Integrity
- Empower staff to respond proactively. Do not let a wound go untended. Empower staff to employ proactive measures to prevent skin problems from developing into a pressure ulcer.
- Engage patients. Educate the patient on how to spot any potential skin problems and encourage him or her to report it to staff immediately.

In the previous case study we consider the efforts at Pocono Medical Center (PMC) to improve its wound care and reduce the incidence of pressure ulcers by not only implementing an effective program for its medical center but also working closely with other health care organizations in the community to improve pressure ulcer prevention communitywide. In another case study, we learn how one home care organization, VNA Hospice of Monroe County—in the same community as Pocono Medical Center and working with the hospital—has worked with its older adult patients to reduce their risk of pressure ulcers and thereby improve older adult patient safety.

Figure 8-2. Wound Care Flow Sheet

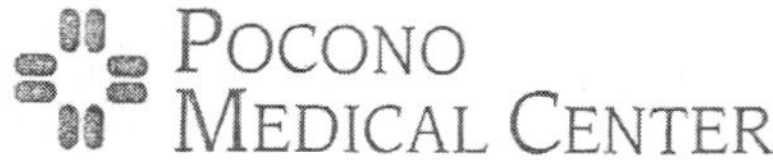

Wound Care Flow Sheet

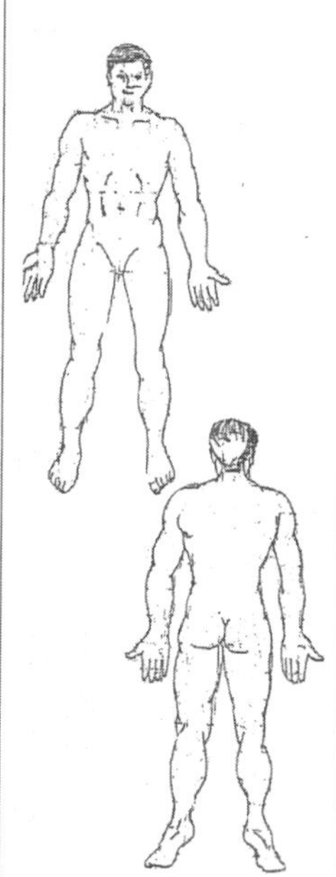

WOUND TYPE

1. Pressure Ulcer Stage ______
2. Diabetic Foot Ulcer
3. Venous Stasis Ulcer
4. Skin Tear
5. Dehisced Wound
6. Trauma
7. Burn
8. Incintinent Dermatitis
9. Other

Mark location on body with letters

SUGGESTED DOCUMENTATION TERMS

WOUND BED

Color– Red, Pink, White, Gray, Black, Tan, Brown

Tissue– Bloody, Pale, Sloughing, Necrotic, Eschar, Granular, Weeping, Healthy

Pain– Yes: 1 (low)–10 (high)

No

DRAINAGE— Absent, Present

Amounts–Scant, Small, Moderate, Large, Copious

Color– Clear, Blood tinged, Yellow, Tan, Purulent, Sanguineous, Green, Gray

Odor– Present, Absent, Foul, Musty

WOUND MARGINS

Edematous, Calloused, Macerated, Clean, Intact, Jagged, Rolled

PERI-WOUND

Pink, White, Red, Pale, Warm, Cool, Blanched, Shiny, Edematous, Indurated

Wound Care Orders: ____________________

____

____

____

Date	Location	Type	Stage	LxWxD in cm.	Wound Bed Color	Pain	Drainage			Wound Margins	Peri-Wound	Dressing		Signature/Title
							Amt	Color	Odor			Intact	Changed	

NS-461F MRC-925
FORMS 5/08

Pilot

Patient Identification

An example of Pocono Medical Center's wound care flow sheet.

Source: *Pocono Medical Center, East Stroudsburg, Pennsylvania. Used with permission.*

Figure 8-3. Interdisciplinary Plan of Care

POCONO MEDICAL CENTER

INTERDISCIPLINARY PLAN OF CARE

Date/ initials	Problem #	Problem	Short Term Goal/Outcome	Interventions	Reviewed/ Revised	Resolve Date/ Initials
	1	Knowledge Deficit Related To:___ ___	❑ Understands ___ ___	❑ Care Notes Distributed and Reviewed ❑		
		PainRelated To:___ ___	❑ Effective Pain Management ❑	❑ Utilize available pain control methods ❑ ❑		
		Safety/Potential for Injury Related To:___ ___	❑ Maintain Safe Environment ❑	❑ Screen for Safety Risks ❑ ❑		
		Actual/potential alteration in skin integrity secondary to pressure ulcer, diabetic ulcer, skin tear, venous stasis ulcer, incontinent dermatitis, other ___ ___	❑ Patient's skin will remain intact without breakdown ❑ Wounds will heal without infection	❑ Assess skin every shift ❑ Position every 2 hrs. ❑ Incontinence checks or toilet PRN ❑ Offer regular hydration ❑ Specialty bed/overlay, cushion boots per physician order		
				❑ ❑ ❑		

Plan of Care Reviewed with Patient and/or Family/Significant Other: ❑ Yes ❑ No, Explain:___
States Understanding: ❑ Yes ❑ No, Needs Reinforcement Date/Initials ___ Date/Initials ___

INITIALS	NAME/TITLE	INITIALS	NAME/TITLE

Pilot

NS-461F MRC-925
FORMS 5/08

Patient Identification

An example of Pocono Medical Center's interdisciplinary plan of action for patients presenting in the emergency department.

Source: *Pocono Medical Center, East Stroudsburg, Pennsylvania. Used with permission.*

Figure 8-4. Staging Guidelines

PRESSURE ULCER NURSING CARE GUIDELINES

	STAGE I/ DEEP TISSUE INJURY OR AT RISK	STAGE II Partial thickness	STAGE III Full thickness	STAGE IV Full thickness	UNSTAGEABLE WOUND
DESCRIPTION	Area is pink, red, and unblanchable or in DTI, purple, mottled, bruised, or blood-filled blister. Skin is intact.	Area is broken, cracked, blistered, or mottled in color.	Area is broken with deep tissue involvement.	Area is broken with muscle/bone involvement. May have extensive drainage. Undermining and tunneling may be present.	Wound bed is covered with eschar or slough (at least 10%–20% of bed).
CONSULTATION	Dietary (If patient east less than 50% of meals for three days or more.)	Dietary	ET Nurse Dietary PT	ET Nurse Dietary PT	ET Nurse Dietary PT surgical consultation
WOUND CLEANSING	Soap and water	Saline (soaked 4x4 gauze or use a 15cc NSS pink vial)	Saline (soaked 4x4 gauze or use a 15cc NSS pink vial)	Saline (soaked 4x4 gauze or use a 15cc NSS pink vial)	Saline (soaked 4x4 gauze or use a 15cc NSS pink vial)
MANAGEMENT/ PRODUCTS DRESSINGS	Protective barriers (i.e., Prevacare, No Sting, Aloe Vera, Calmoseptine, Xenaderm or other moisture barrier cream)	Dry or moderately exudating wounds: 1. Moisture barrier gel to open areas (e.g., Tegaderm Hydrogel, Carrington Gel, or Xenaderm). 2. Cover with a hydrocolloid dressing (e.g., Extra Thin DuoDerm, CGF) or Adherent Silicone (Mepilex). 3. Change every 3–5 days & PRN. Heavily exudating wounds 1. Alignate dressing (i.e., Kalstat or Sorbsan) OR Mesalt OR Foam. 2. Change dressing PRN. Beefy wound beds 1. Collagen Dressing (Prisma) change every 48 hours initially, then every 72 hours thereafter. Moisten if dry. 2. Cover with secondary dressing.	Dry or moderately exudating wounds: Choices: 1. Moist-to-moist saline dressing every day. [NO LONGER RECOMMENDED] OR 2. Moisture barrier gel as needed, cover with hydrocolloid dressing or silicone dressing. a. Change every 3–5 days & PRN. OR Heavily exudating wounds 1. Calcium alginate dressing (e.g., Kalstat or Sorbsan) OR Silicone dressing (Mepilex). 2. Cover with gauze dressing. 3. Change dressing PRN OR VAC (see standing orders)	Dry or moderately exudating wounds: Choices: 1. Moist-to-moist saline dressing every day. [NO LONGER RECOMMENDED] OR 2. Moisture barrier gel as needed, cover with hydrocolloid dressing or silicone dressing. a. Change every 3–5 days & PRN. OR Heavily exudating wounds 1. Calcium alginate dressing (e.g., Kalstat or Sorbsan) OR Silicone dressing (Mepilex). 2. Cover with gauze dressing. 3. Change dressing PRN OR VAC (see standing orders)	Debridement method as per physician order: Choices: 1. Mechanical. a. Moist-to-moist Saline every day (NO LONGER RECOMMENDED). 2. Chemical. a. Enzymatic (enzyme ointment; e.g., Santyl). 3. Autolytic. a. Hyro-colloid dressings. b. Hypergel 4. Surgical. a. Post-debridement wound dressing as per MD (surgeon's) order. OR b. VAC (see standing orders).
BEDS/SUPPORT SURFACES	1. Air overlay 2.. Versa 3. Zone-Air 4. Waffle overlay	1. Versa 2.. Air/Foam Combo (Zone-Air) 3. Eclipse 4. Waffle overlay	1.. Air/Foam Combo (Zone-Air) 2. Eclipse 3. Versa 4. Rite Hite	1.. Air/Foam Combo (Zone-Air) 2. Eclipse 3. Versa 4. Rite Hite	*Rite Hite OR WORST CASE Clinitron

An example of Pocono Medical Center's pressure ulcer nursing care guidelines.

Source: *Pocono Medical Center, East Stroudsburg, Pennsylvania. Used with permission.*

Figure 8-5. Skin Management

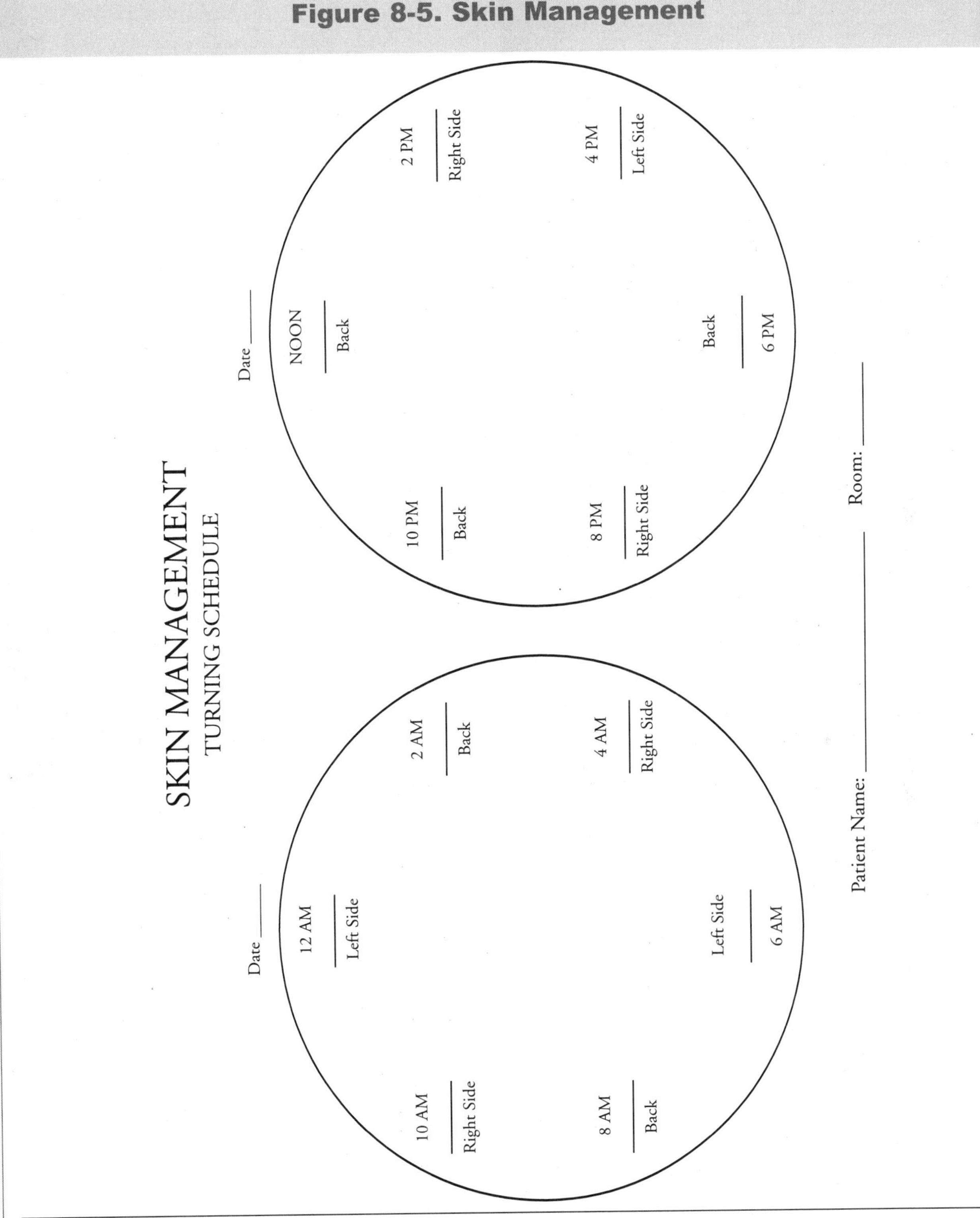

An example of Pocono Medical Center's turning schedule for the management of patients' skin for pressure ulcers.

Source: *Pocono Medical Center, East Stroudsburg, Pennsylvania. Used with permission.*

CASE STUDY

Spotlight on Improvement: VNA Hospice of Monroe County's Comprehensive Assessment Approach for Older Adult Patients

For the VNA Hospice of Monroe County, located in East Stroudsburg, Pennsylvania, a comprehensive and ongoing assessment of home care–based older adult patients goes without saying. "All of our patients are given a robust assessment on admission, even including an assessment of any potential safety and falls risks," explains Marie Dooner, R.N., performance improvement nurse, VNA Hospice of Monroe County.

Older Adult Patient Assessments in Home Care

VNA Hospice also does a medication assessment to see if the patient is cognitively fit to provide his or her own medications and a foot assessment. They also conduct medication reconciliation on admission. Catherine Koch, a certified wound ostomy and continence nurse who has additional expertise in home care (*see* the Spotlight on Improvement, pages 103–105), often performs the admissions and assessments for VNA Hospice. Her expertise in skin assessment and wound care has proven valuable to the agency in establishing a framework of care for those patients who are at high risk for pressure ulcers.

"In relation to any safety assessment that a nurse conducts, the patient gets a copy of the nurse's findings," says Dooner. "If the nurse finds that the patient or the patient's caregivers are not capable of taking care of any problem, then social services is approached. Then we have them come and do an evaluation of the home for safety and to make sure that the home is safe for them to be served in."

Dooner explains that their approach to assessment and care planning is built on compliance guidance from both The Joint Commission and the CMS. "Everything we do is geared toward compliance with high standards for patient safety," Dooner notes.

Staff Education

Achieving success requires good staff education, notes Nancy Bellissimo, performance improvement nurse, VNA Hospice of Monroe County. "As long as you have an education program geared toward keeping your staff and workers informed in best practices in home care, then you've won half the battle," she explains.

VA Hospice uses ongoing in-service education throughout the year, and although it has focused on a range of issues facing its patients, for older adult patients some training has included such topics as falling, various problems for specific older adult patients, and medication.

One practical approach to training that has been employed by VNA Hospice is the use of voice mail to leave educational messages. Bellissimo leaves messages with education information so that staff can listen at their leisure and convenience. Some staff prefer not to use the voice mail system, so VNA Hospice provides follow-up education as well.

Benefiting from Staff Skills

In regard to skin assessment and wound care for the home care patients, Dooner notes that Koch's expertise and work with the agency, along with her work at the hospital, has made a big difference in such areas as wound care competence. Having a staff at the agency with specialized skills is a real asset, she says.

An important aspect of wound care and skin assessment is the performance of a full body system assessment. "Every time one of our nurses goes to visit that patient, she does a full body system assessment, so she's able to determine whether a patient's condition is worsening or [improving],"

At-a-Glance

About the home care organization: The Visiting Nurses Association (VNA) Hospice of Monroe County, located in East Stroudsburg, Pennsylvania, provides home care and hospice services in the East Stroudsburg region.

About the improvement: The VNA conducts a robust and ongoing assessment process for its older adult patients, particularly in such areas as falls risk and wound assessment.

notes Dooner. "Her assessment abilities help ward off a lot of problems." Partnered with the assessment is the agency's electronic system that triggers a response if the skin assessment points to a deterioration in the patient so the agency can respond with appropriate wound care.

But above all, the unique nature of home care means that a nurse can make a significant difference in older adult patient safety. "The nurse has an important role in home care to observe and see what issues may exist," Dooner notes.

Patient Education

Patient education is another focus for the agency. "Our nurses and therapists have various forms and handouts to give to the patient," Bellissimo says. "There is a hands-on, ongoing, verbal teaching program, which is documented during each visit."

In all, VNA Hospice's assessment is time consuming but worth the work. "We ask a lot of our nurses and therapists, it takes over an hour to do it, but it's an important element of our patient safety efforts," Bellissimo notes.

Tips for Improvement

Bellissimo and Dooner share the following recommendations for other home care agencies working to improve older adult patient safety efforts.

For a new agency or someone new to home care, Dooner and Bellissimo suggest that they avail themselves of all the resources open to them—from such agencies as the CMS or The Joint Commission.

To have a good agency and deliver good care, you must adhere to the standards and regulations. Only then are you ready to deliver good care and ensure patient safety.

No one can be fully successful with patient safety and good patient care without help. It comes from the combined minds and efforts of many people.

Be open to mentoring others, share your knowledge, and be patient with the process.

With an effective assessment process and success in keeping its patients well educated and safe, VNA Hospice has become a mentor to other newer home care agencies. This kind of collaboration and support is the kind of opportunity that staff at VNA Hospice relish. They also look forward to the collaborative work ahead in the community for pressure ulcer reductions by participating on the skin team with PMC (*see* the Spotlight on Improvement on page 103–105). This kind of work is seen by VNA Hospice as helping the organization meet its goals for ensuring that its patients are safe and well cared for.

Incontinence Issues

Incontinence—both urinary and fecal—affects a significant number of older adult patients. Although aging can increase the incidence of incontinence, other older adult patient safety risks can also cause it: infection, polypharmacy, and decreased cognitive function.[10] As one study notes, "The presence of chronic incontinence can produce a vicious cycle of skin damage and inflammation because of the loss of cutaneous integrity."[10]

Related to skin care and pressure ulcer prevention, effectively managing incontinence can help prevent skin problems, which could lead to pressure ulcers. In addition, the use of catheters in urinary incontinence sufferers can cause urinary tract infections, a patient safety concern. Good clinical management of incontinence along with regular assessments to ensure that there are no skin problems can help prevent other risk factors for older adult patients and improve quality of life.

Conclusion

Older adult patients face special risks that organizations need to be aware of and assess for in an ongoing manner. One particular area is in relation to developing pressure ulcers, for which older adult patients are at higher risk. As such, effectively managing incontinence and wounds and careful skin assessments can help prevent pressure ulcers. Ensuring that staff and the organization understand and can assess for the risk factors associated with pressure ulcers can go a long way toward helping mitigate and prevent their occurrence.

This entire publication has been devoted to the special needs and concerns for ensuring the safety of older adult patients. Although it is never possible to guarantee that no patient will ever experience an adverse event or to ensure that all systems and processes in a health care organization will be error proof, systematic efforts to design systems and processes that can help reduce the chances of sentinel events can make a significant difference. Many of the issues raised and strategies included in this publication point to one underlying yet important issue for any health care organization to pursue in its older adult patient safety efforts, indeed in any kind of patient safety work: the need for an organizational culture oriented toward safety. This kind of culture is one where, as the Institute for Healthcare Improvement states, "People are not merely encouraged to work toward change, they take action when it is needed."[11]

Ensuring that older adult patients, a vulnerable population that can be more susceptible to ill health, are safe requires action on the part of staff: empowerment to act when needed and support from the organization to provide the best quality safe care to the patients that it serves. This kind of culture, a culture of safety, can help sustain patient safety efforts for the long term. And with a growing aging population facing complex health care concerns and adding an increasing burden to health care systems around the world, now is the time for organizations to work toward building and sustaining a culture of safety.

References

1. Lynn J., et al.: Collaborative clinical quality improvement for pressure ulcers in nursing homes. *J Am Geriatr Soc* 55:1663–1669, 2007.
2. Cuddigan J., Berlowitz D.R., Ayello E.A.: *Pressure ulcers in America: prevalence, incidence, and implications for the future.* Reston, VA: National Pressure Ulcer Advisory Panel, 2001.
3. Pope, C.: The act of pressure ulcer prevention. *Mater Manag Health Care* 10:18–22, 2008.
4. Tannen A., et al.: Explaining the national differences in pressure ulcer prevalence between the Netherlands and Germany—Adjusted for personal risk factors and institutional quality indicators. *J Eval Clin Pract* 15:85–90, Feb. 2009.
5. Lyder C.H., Ayello E.A.: Pressure ulcers: A patient safety issue. In *Patient Safety and Quality: An Evidence-Based Handbook for Nurses.* AHRQ: http://www.ahrq.gov/qual/nurseshdbk/ (accessed Feb. 19, 2009).
6. American Medical Directors Association: *AMDA Pressure Ulcer Clinical Guidelines.* Colombia, MD: AMDA, 2007.
7. McInerney J.A.: Reducing hospital-acquired pressure ulcer prevalence through a focused prevention program. *J Wound Care* pp. 75–78, Feb. 2008.
8. Vu T., et al.: Cost-effectiveness of multidisciplinary wound care in nursing homes. *Fam Pract* 24:372–379, 2007.
9. Centers for Medicare and Medicaid Services: Tag F-314 pressure ulcers. (Revised.) *Guidance for Surveyors in Long Term Care.* http://www.cms.hhs.gov/SurveyCertificationGenInfo/downloads/SCLetter05-17.pdf (accessed Mar. 23, 2009).
10. Farage M.A., et al.: Incontinence in the aged: Contact dermatitis and other cutaneous consequences. *Contact Dermatitis* 57:211–217, 2007.
11. Institute for Healthcare Improvement: http://www.ihi.org/IHI/Topics/PatientSafety/MedicationSystems/Changes/Develop+a+Culture+of+Safety.htm (accessed Mar. 23, 2009).

Appendix

Resources for Older Adults

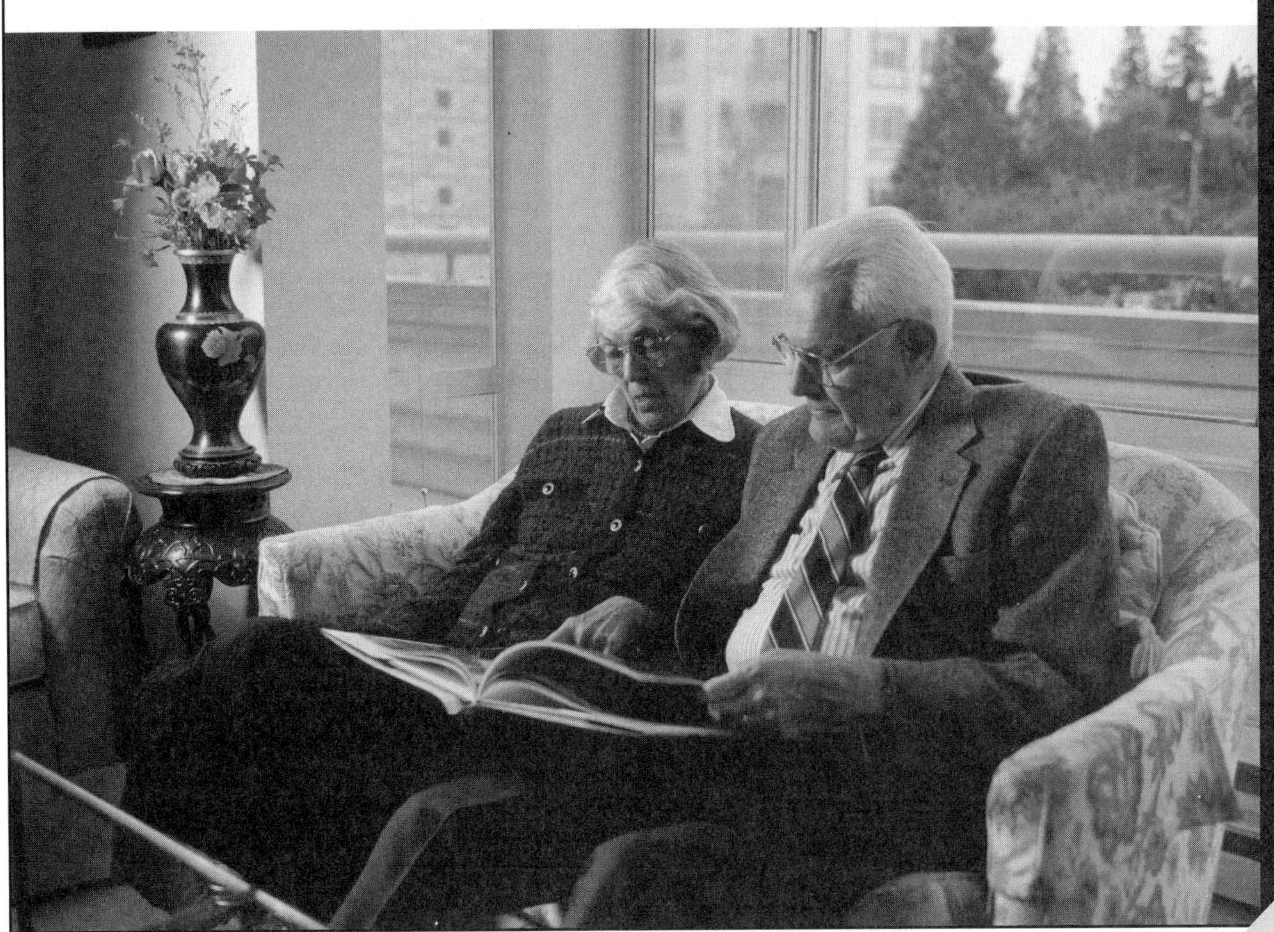

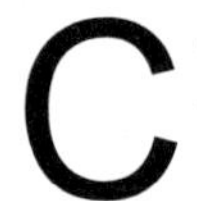

Contained in this appendix are some resources for the geriatric population listed by topic.

Dementia

Age Page: Patient- and family-oriented information on cognitive issues and dementia. http://www.nia.nih.gov/healthinformation/publications/forgetfulness.htm

American Association for Geriatric Psychiatry (AAGP): An organization that advocates for the mental health needs of the elderly. http://www.aagpgpa.org

American Association of Retired Persons (AARP):
http://www.aarp.org

American Geriatrics Society:
http://www.americangeriatrics.org

Alzheimer's Disease Education and Referral (ADEAR) Center: A service of the National Institute on Aging, the ADEAR Center offers information and publications in English and Spanish for families and caregivers on diagnosis, treatment, patient care, caregiver needs, long term care, and research related to dementia.
P.O. Box 8250, Silver Spring, MD 20907-8250, 800-438-4380 (toll-free), http://www.nia.nih.gov/Alzheimers

Alzheimer's Association:
225 North Michigan Avenue, Floor 17, Chicago, IL 60601-7633, 800-272-3900 (toll-free), 866-403-3073 (TDD/toll-free), http://www.alz.org

Alzheimer's Association Fact Sheets and Brochures:
http://www.alz.org/alzheimers_disease_publications.asp

Eldercare Locator:
800-677-1116 (toll-free), http://www.eldercare.gov

Depression and Suicide

National Institute on Aging: The National Institute on Aging provides patient- and family-specific information on depression and suicide risk at http://www.nia.nih.gov/healthinformation/publications/depression.htm. It also includes the following resources for organizations and patients on depression and suicide risk:

American Association for Geriatric Psychiatry:
7910 Woodmont Avenue, Suite 1050, Bethesda, MD 20814-3004, 301-654-7850, http://www.aagpgpa.org

American Psychological Association:
750 First Street, NE, Washington, DC 20002-4242, 800-374-2721 (toll-free), 202-336-6123 (TDD/TTY), http://www.apa.org

Depression and Bipolar Support Alliance:
730 North Franklin Street, Suite 501, Chicago, IL 60610-7224, 800-826-3632 (toll-free)
http://www.dbsalliance.org

Mental Health America:
2000 North Beauregard Street, 6th Floor, Alexandria, VA 22311, 800-969-6642 (toll-free), 800-433-5959 (TTY/toll-free), http://www.nmha.org

National Alliance on Mental Illness:
Colonial Place Three, 2107 Wilson Boulevard, Suite 300, Arlington, VA 22201-3042, 800-950-6264 (toll-free), http://www.nami.org

National Institute of Mental Health:
6001 Executive Boulevard, Room 8184, MSC 9663, Bethesda, MD 20892-9663, 866-615-6464 (for publications/toll-free), 866-415-8951 (TTY/toll-free), http://www.nimh.nih.gov

National Suicide Prevention Lifeline:
800-273-8255 (toll-free, 24 hours a day), 800-799-4889 (TTY)

Elder Abuse

Regulatory/Authoritative Sites

American Geriatrics Society: Guidelines and Position Statements: http://www.americangeriatrics.org/products/positionpapers/

American Medical Directors Association (AMDA):
Resource Library: http://amda.com

Elder Abuse information:
http://www.nlm.nih.gov/medlineplus/elderabuse.html

Gerontological Society of America: http://www.geron.org

National Center on Elder Abuse (NCEA): http://www.ncea.aoa.gov

National Conference of Gerontological Nurse Practitioners: http://www.gapna.org

National Gerontological Nursing Association: http://www.ngna.org

United States Department of Health & Human Services: http://www.hhs.gov

Government Information Agencies

Administration on Aging: http://www.aoa.gov

American Bar Association Commission on Law and Aging: http://www.abanet.org/elderly

Clearinghouse on Abuse and Neglect of the Elderly: http://www.cane.udel.edu/

Environmental Protection Agency: Includes a program as an initiative designed to study and prioritize the environmental health risks seniors face. Information about this evolving research agenda is available from the Web site: http://www.epa.gov/aging

National Association of State Units on Aging: http://www.nasua.org/

National Adult Protective Services Association: http://www.apsnetwork.org/

National Committee for the Prevention of Elder Abuse: http://www.preventelderabuse.org

National Guideline Clearinghouse/Agency for Healthcare Research and Quality: http://www.guideline.gov/summary/summary.aspx?doc_id=6829&nbr=4196&string=elder+AND+abuse

National Institute on Aging: The NIA conducts and supports biomedical, social, and behavioral research; provides research training; and disseminates research findings and health information on aging processes, diseases, and other special problems and needs of older people. http://www.nia.nih.gov

United States Census: *The Older Population in the United States* (March 1999), a PDF document from the U.S. Census Bureau Current Population Reports http://www.census.gov/prod/2003pubs/p20-546.pdf

United States Department of Health & Human Services: http://www.hhs.gov/aging/index.shtml

United States Department of Health and Human Services, HealthFinder: A gateway to consumer health and human services information. Vast selection of hot topics and specifically-tailored links for health professionals, such as clinical trials and self-help groups. http://www.healthfinder.org

White House Conference on Aging (2005): http://www.whcoa.gov

Patient and Family Resources

Age Page: Crime and Older People: http://www.nia.nih.gov/HealthInformation/Publications/crime.htm

American Geriatrics Society: *Aging in the Know* http://www.healthinaging.org/agingintheknow

Elder abuse information: http://www.nlm.nih.gov/medlineplus/elderabuse.html

National Citizen's Coalition for Nursing Home Reform: http://www.nccnhr.org/default.cfm

National Institutes of Health: *Health Information* http://health.nih.gov

National Long Term Care Ombudsman Resource Center: http://www.ltcombudsman.org

United States Department of Health & Human Services, Centers for Disease Control and Prevention: http://www.cdc.gov

U.S. National Library of Medicine and National Institutes of Health: Medline Plus Links to multiple governmental, private, and professional Web site. http://www.nlm.nih.gov/medlineplus

Falls and Falls Prevention

AgePage, Falls: http://www.nia.nih.gov/HealthInformation/Publications/falls.htm

American Tai Chi Association: Information about tai chi, where to find a class nationwide, instruction books, and DVDs. http://www.americantaichi.org

Centers for Disease Control and Prevention Injury Center: How to prevent falls, tips for fall-proofing your home. http://www.cdc.gov/ncipc/duip/preventadultfalls.htm

Department of Health and Human Services, Centers for Disease Control and Prevention (CDC): Home Page. http://www.cdc.gov

Falls: *NIH Institute and Center Resources.* http://health.nih.gov/result.asp/252

Lighthouse International: Leading resource worldwide on vision impairment and vision rehabilitation. http://www.lighthouse.org

National Center for Injury Prevention and Control: *What You Can Do to Prevent Falls: Senior Falls: A Toolkit to Prevent Falls.* http://www.cdc.gov/ncipc/pub-res/toolkit/WhatYouCanDoToPreventFalls.htm

National Council on Aging: Checklists, questionnaires, and fact sheet on preventing falls. http://www.healthyagingprograms.org/content.asp?sectionid=69

National Institutes of Health (NIH): *Health Information.*
Home Page: http://health.nih.gov
Seniors' Health: http://health.nih.gov/search.asp/27

National Osteoporosis Foundation: Patient information on fall prevention. http://www.nof.org/patientinfo/fall_prevention.htm

Other resources on fall prevention and aging: http://www.temple.edu/older_adult/agresou.htm

Senior Health at the National Institutes of Health: Senior-friendly Web pages about balance. http://nihseniorhealth.gov/balanceproblems/aboutbalanceproblems/02.html

Temple University: The Fall Prevention Project In-Home Safety Check. http://www.temple.edu/older_adult/IHSCEng.htm

United States Department of Health and Human Services. http://www.hhs.gov

U.S. National Library of Medicine and National Institutes of Health: Medline Plus Links to multiple governmental, private, and professional Web sites. http://www.nlm.nih.gov/medlineplus

Health and Aging

American Health Care Association (AHCA): http://www.ahcancal.org

American Society on Aging: Web site includes training opportunities, information on publications, and a calendar of conference events on aging. http://www.asaging.org/index.cfm

Association for Gerontology in Higher Education: An educational unit of the Gerontological Society of America, promoting education and training in the field of aging. http://www.aghe.org

British Society of Gerontology: http://www.britishgerontology.org

Canadian Association on Gerontology: http://www.cagacg.ca

Gerontological Society of America: http://www.geron.org

Global Action on Aging: http://www.globalaging.org/

Healthy Ageing: An EU-funded project from 2004–2007. http://www.healthyageing.nu

National Academy on an Aging Society: A nonpartisan, policy institute that fosters critical thinking about the implications of an aging society. http://www.agingsociety.org

National Association of Professional Geriatric Care Managers: http://www.caremanager.org

National Hispanic Council on Aging: In addition to descriptions of programs and projects, this organization provides a legislative update. http://www.nhcoa.org

National Institute on Aging Information Center: P.O. Box 8057, Gaithersburg, MD 20898-8057, 800-222-2225 (toll-free), 800-222-4225 (TTY/toll-free), http://www.nia.nih.gov or http://www.nia.nih.gov/Espanol

NIH SeniorHealth: A senior-friendly Web site from the National Institute on Aging and the National Library of Medicine. This Web site has health information for older adults. Special features make it simple to use. For example, you can click on a button to have the text read out loud or to make the type larger. http://www.nihseniorhealth.gov

Services and Advocacy for Gay, Lesbian, Bisexual & Transgender Elders: http://www.sageusa.org

United Nations Programme on Ageing: http://www.un.org/esa/socdev/ageing/

World Health Organization (WHO): http://www.who.int/topics/ageing/en

Medication Management

Age Page, Medications: http://www.nia.nih.gov/HealthInformation/Publications/medicines.htm http://www.nia.nih.gov/HealthInformation/Publications/SafeUseMeds

ConsultGeriRN.org: Geriatric *Nursing Practice: Medication.* http://www.consultgerirn.org/topics/medication/want_to_know_more

Geriatric Patient Safety Initiative: http://www.feinberg.northwestern.edu/ihs/program-centers/cps/gps1.html

USP: *Medication Errors Involving Geriatric Patients.* http://www.usp.org/pdf/EN/patientSafety/drugSafetyReview2004-01-26.pdf

Other Sites of Interest

American Psychological Association Office on Aging: http://www.apa.org/pi/aging

Andrus Gerontology Library at the University of Southern California: Links to bibliographies on specific subtopics in gerontology, as well as research guides. http://www.usc.edu/libraries/locations/gerontology

CSWE National Center for Gerontological Social Work Education: A new site that intends to present gerontological teaching resources and curricular ideas. http://depts.washington.edu/geroctr

ElderWeb: A research site for both professionals and family members looking for information on eldercare and long term care. Includes links to information on legal, financial, medical, and housing issues, as well as policy, research, and statistics. http://www.elderweb.com/home

Michigan eLibrary—Aging Web page: http://melweb.mlcnet.org/viewtopic.jsp?id=817&pathid=1462

UK Department for Work and Pensions: http://dwp.gov.uk/agepositive

University of Michigan Geriatrics Center: Includes links to the Turner Geriatric Clinical. http://www.med.umich.edu/geriatrics/TurnerGeriatricClinic/primarycare.htm

University of Michigan Institute of Gerontology: http://www.iog.umich.edu

Urban Institute—Retirement Policy: Assesses how current retirement policies, demographic trends, and private sector practices affect the well-being of older Americans and the economy. The project also analyzes proposed retirement policies, with a focus on both the income and health needs of the elderly. http://www.urban.org/retirement_policy/index.cfm

Wayne State University Institute of Gerontology: http://www.iog.wayne.edu

Index

B

C

D

E

F

R

S